Subtotal Thyroidectomy

Single Surgical Procedures 5

A Colour Atlas of

Subtotal Thyroidectomy

Peter H. Dickinson

W DE G

Walter de Gruyter · Berlin · New York 1984

Peter H. Dickinson MB, BS (Dunelm) MSc (Surgery, Illinois), FRCS (England), FRCS (Edin.); Senior Consultant Surgeon, Royal Victory Infirmacy, Newcastle upon Tyne; Lecturer in Clinical Surgery, The Medical School, University of Newcastle upon Tyne

Original Publishers: Wolfe Medical Publications Ltd., · London
Exclusive co-publishers for the Federal Republic of Germany and Austria: Walter de Gruyter & Co., Genthiner Strasse 13, D-1000 Berlin 30. 1984.

Printed by Royal Smeets Offset b.v., Weert, Netherlands

Cover design: Rudolf Hübler

General Editor, Wolfe Surgical Atlases:
William F. Walker, DSc, ChM, FRCS (Eng.), FRCS (Edin.), FRS (Edin.)

CIP-Kurztitelaufnahme der Deutschen Bibliothek

Dickinson, Peter H.:
A colour atlas of subtotal thyroidectomy / Peter H. Dickinson. -
Berlin; New York: de Gruyter, 1984.
(Single surgical procedures; 5)
ISBN 3-11-010015-0
ISBN 3-11-010014-2 (Subskr.-Pr.)
NE: GT

Contents

Introduction

Subtotal thyroidectomy is the standard operative procedure in the surgical treatment of thyrotoxicosis. Medical treatment of thyrotoxicosis may be by drug therapy or radioiodine. The choice of treatment, medical or surgical, will vary with the individual patient, the doctor and the clinical circumstances.

This Atlas is concerned solely with the operation of subtotal thyroidectomy for thyrotoxicosis. Nevertheless, mention must be made of drug therapy because it has an essential role to play in the preparation of the patient for surgery; no patient is operated upon while still toxic, but is first rendered euthyroid by an antithyroid drug such as carbimazole.

The diagnosis of thyrotoxicosis is made on clinical grounds and confirmed by laboratory investigations, which may also help to determine the cause of the hyperthyroidism. Commonly employed tests are measurement of the level of thyroid hormones (T4 and T3) in the blood which have now replaced the in vivo thyroid uptake of isotopes of iodine or pertechnetate. Thyroid isotope scanning using ^{99m}Tc or ^{123}I, can help to distinguish between a diffuse and a nodular goitre. In most cases of Graves' disease autoantibodies to thyroid components are present and are determined by standard immunological investigation.

Once the diagnosis of thyrotoxicosis has been established the aim of treatment is to reduce the level of thyroid hormone in the blood. This is done initially with one of the antithyroid drugs. Carbimazole is commonly used in the UK (45 mg daily in divided dosage). The patient usually becomes euthyroid in four to six weeks, the clinical improvement being confirmed by estimation of the blood level of T4 and TSH. When the patient is euthyroid the drug dose is reduced to a maintenance level (approximately half the initial dosage) unless the patient has been chosen for surgical treatment, when the initial dose is maintained up to the time of operation.

There is the possibility that during drug therapy the thyroid gland will become larger and more vascular, making surgery more difficult. The likelihood of this happening may be reduced by the administration of thyroxine (100–200 mcg/day) for at least three weeks before operation. All drugs are discontinued the day before operation. Some clinicians now favour the use of propanalol as the sole therapy before thyroidectomy.

Surgical treatment is designed to render permanent the reduction of thyroid hormone in the blood achieved by drug therapy. The basis of the operation of subtotal thyroidectomy is to remove sufficient thyroid tissue to make this possible. A much discussed problem is how much gland should be removed or, alternatively, how large or small should the gland remnants be. The amount of thyroid tissue which is left behind will obviously be governed to some extent by the original size of the gland and the quality of the remaining tissue; some thyroid glands may contain degenerative nodules or be affected by autoimmune thyroiditis, remnants of such glands will need to be larger. The size of the remnants in relation to the incidence of postoperative hypothyroidism or hyperthyroidism has, however, been shown not to be critical.

The method of subtotal thyroidectomy to be described in this Atlas is the one used routinely by the author. Obviously, variations in technique are used by individual thyroid surgeons. For example, the question of whether or not the infrahyoid muscles should be divided is much discussed; the author prefers not to divide them routinely; other surgeons believe they should always be divided, particularly to provide better access to the posterolateral areas of the thyroid lobes.

In over 1,000 thyroidectomies, however, the author has found division of the strap muscles to be necessary in only a few; but when the surgeon is inexperienced and the goitre large it may be wiser to divide the muscles until more experience is gained. The author prefers, if possible, to identify the recurrent laryngeal nerves and the parathyroid glands. The recurrent laryngeal nerves are usually easy to identify either by sight or feel, but the parathyroid glands present greater difficulty because they are variable in number, position and colour and they may have a covering of fat. Usually they are seen as small brown/yellow structures, the upper lying on the posterolateral aspect of the upper part of the thyroid and the lower near the branches of the inferior thyroid artery as they enter the thyroid gland. The normal brown/yellow colour is easily altered by even gentle handling and they may then be seen as dark-red or plum-coloured structures.

When the parathyroid glands are not found quickly there is no need to go to extreme lengths to identify them, because they can be damaged easily by mobilisation. If the parathyroid glands are not identified early the search should be abandoned; the same applies to the recurrent laryngeal nerves.

Positioning of patient, skin incision, and exposure of thyroid gland

1
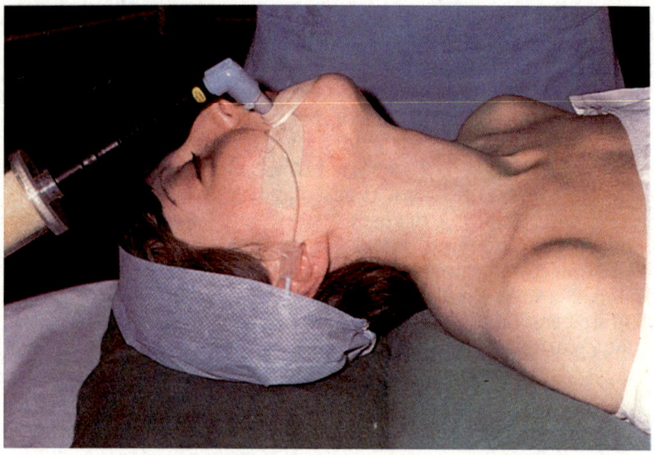

2
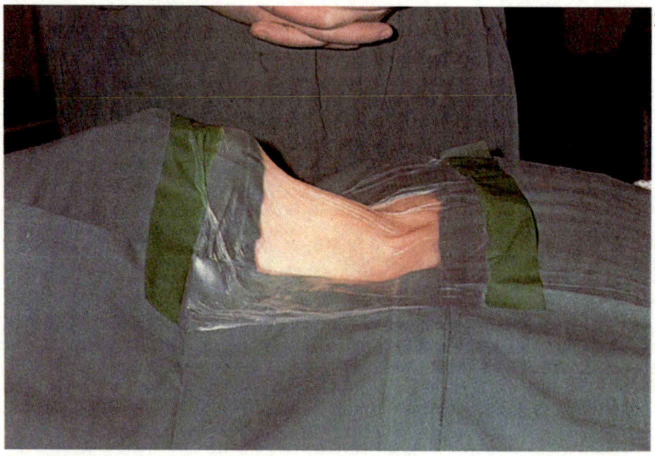

1 Position of patient. The patient is placed on the operating table with the neck well extended. This may be achieved by the two-pillow technique. The two pillows are stepped as shown, with the shoulders positioned where the two pillows overlap. The head rests comfortably on the single pillow above the overlap.

2 Towel application. Towels are applied in rectangular fashion around the operation field and held in position by towel clips. A plastic adhesive membrane (Op-Site) is then placed on the skin and over the towel edges.

3 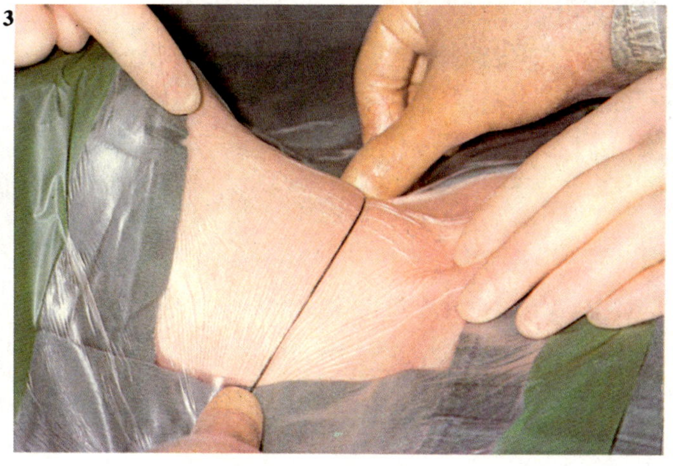

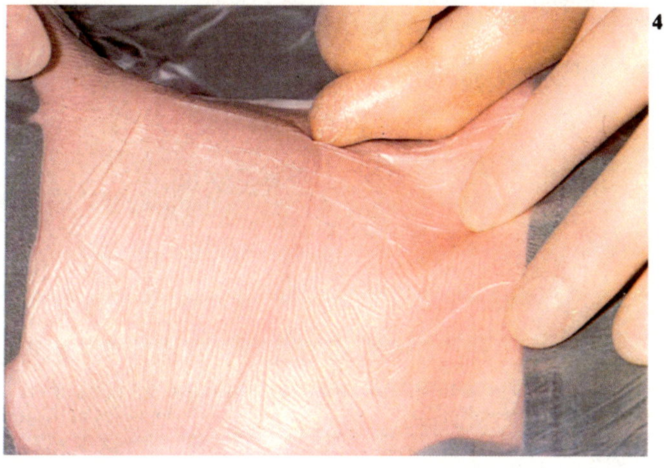 4

3 Skin incision siting. The siting of the skin incision is important; a badly positioned scar will be unsightly. The line of the skin incision is marked out by a thread which indents the skin. The assistant places one index finger on the point of the chin and the other on the suprasternal notch to assist accurate positioning of the thread.

4 Ensuring a horizontal incision line. The resulting transverse indentation is shown and its position is checked by the 'rule of thumb'; the distal phalanx of the operator's thumb measures the distance of the incision line from the clavicle on each side of the neck. Equal measurements ensure that the incision will be horizontal.

5

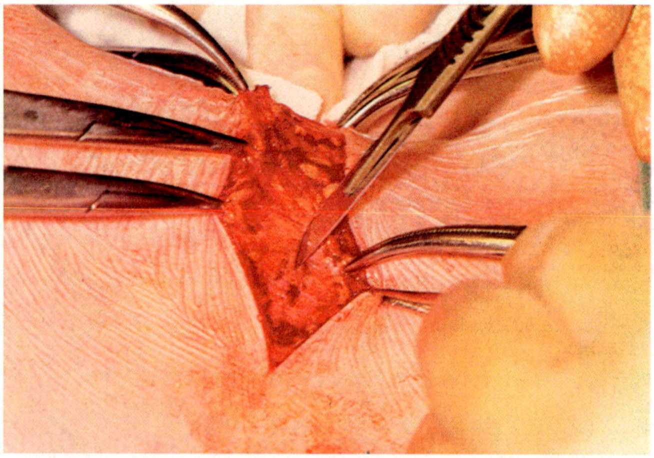

6

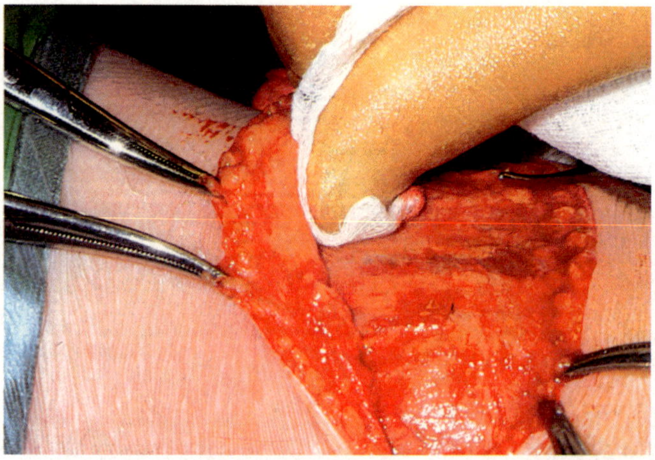

5 Deepening skin incision. The skin incision is deepened through the superficial fascia and platysma muscle. Upper and lower flaps of skin, fascia and platysma muscle are then raised from the underlying strap muscles.

6 Raising skin-flaps. The flaps may be fashioned by blunt dissection using a gauze mop.

7 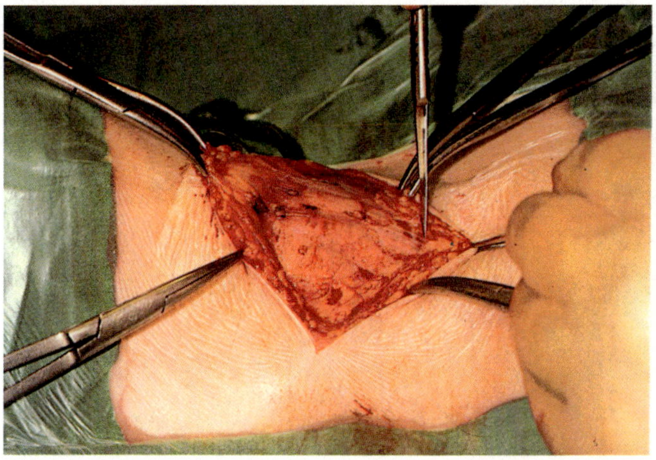

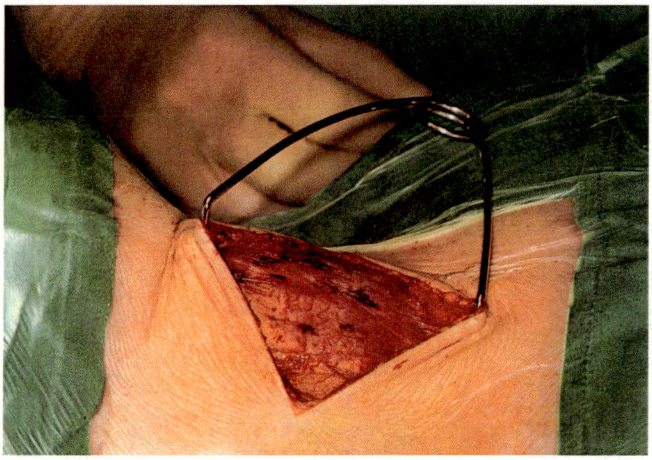 8

7 **Raising skin-flaps.** The skin-flaps may be also raised by knife dissection. Usually a combination of blunt dissection and knife dissection techniques are used. Small bleeding points are sealed by diathermy. Larger vessels are ligated. Throughout the operation the author uses non-absorbable material for ligatures; some surgeons prefer catgut.

8 **Holding back flaps.** The flaps are held back by a single Sloane's spring retractor.

9

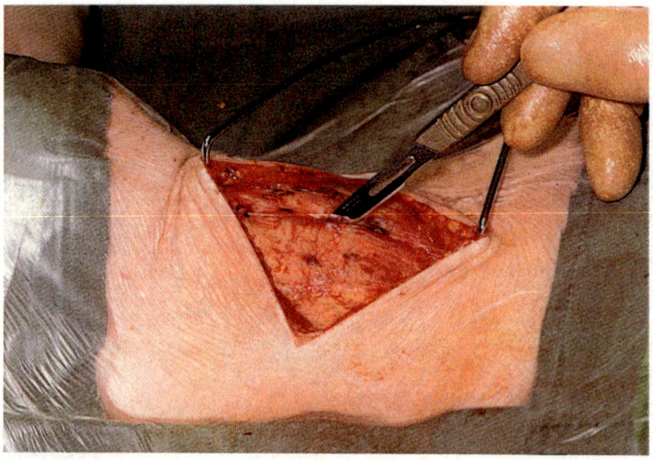

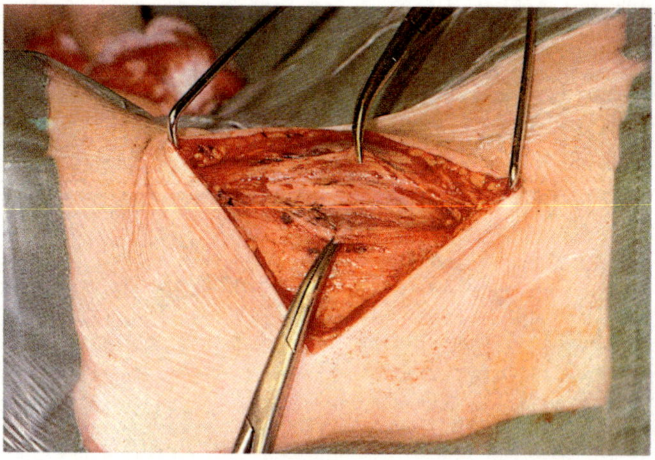

10

9 Separation of strap muscles. A vertical incision is made between the strap muscles in the midline.

10 Exposure of isthmus of thyroid gland. The medial edges of the strap muscles are here held apart revealing the isthmus of the thyroid gland.

Mobilisation of left thyroid lobe

11 Choice of lobe. The areolar tissue deep to the strap muscles is separated to open up the plane between the strap muscles and the capsule of the left lobe of the thyroid gland. The choice of which thyroid lobe to expose first is an individual one, as is the side on which the surgeon stands. The author's preference is to stand on the side opposite to the lobe being mobilised.

All photographs in this Atlas are taken from the same side of the patient as the surgeon is standing, unless otherwise stated.

11

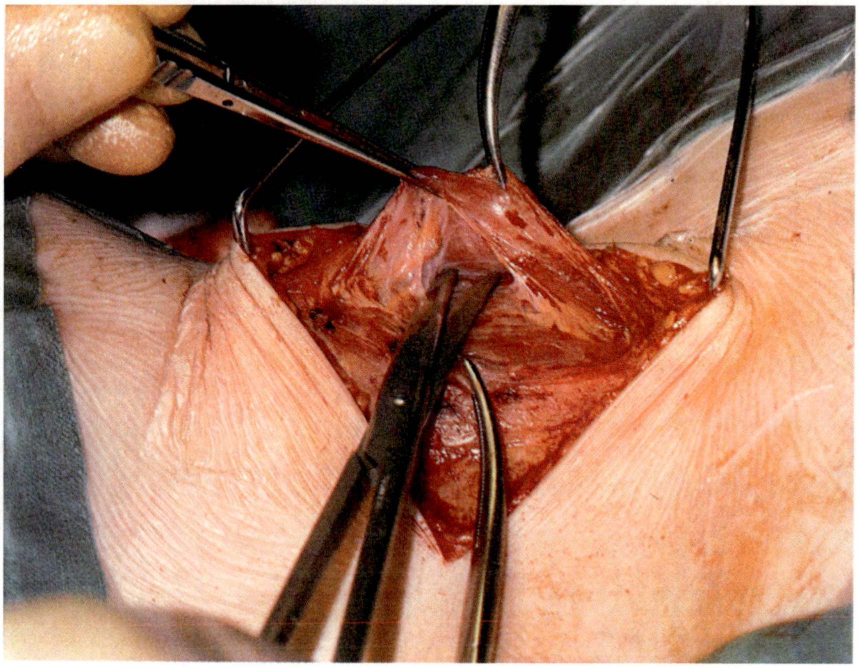

12 Middle thyroid vein. The left thyroid lobe is grasped in Lahey gland-holding forceps and pulled medially. The middle thyroid vein (which can vary considerably in size and position) is sought. It is shown here held up by dissecting forceps in its classic position running laterally from the middle of the thyroid lobe to cross the common carotid artery and enter the internal jugular vein.

12

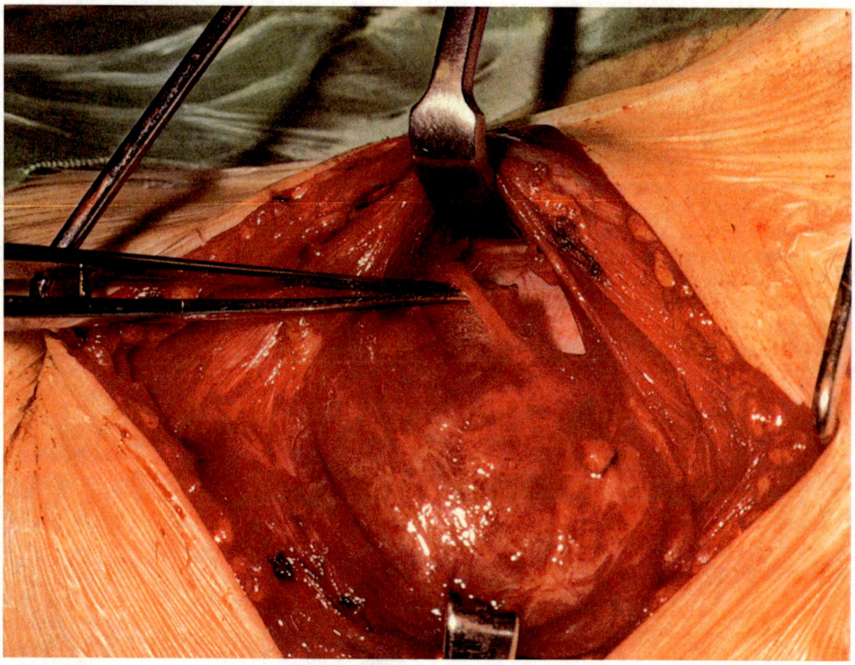

13 Division and ligation of middle thyroid vein. The middle thyroid vein is secured between two artery forceps, divided and ligated. Access to the posterolateral aspect of the lobe is now possible.

13

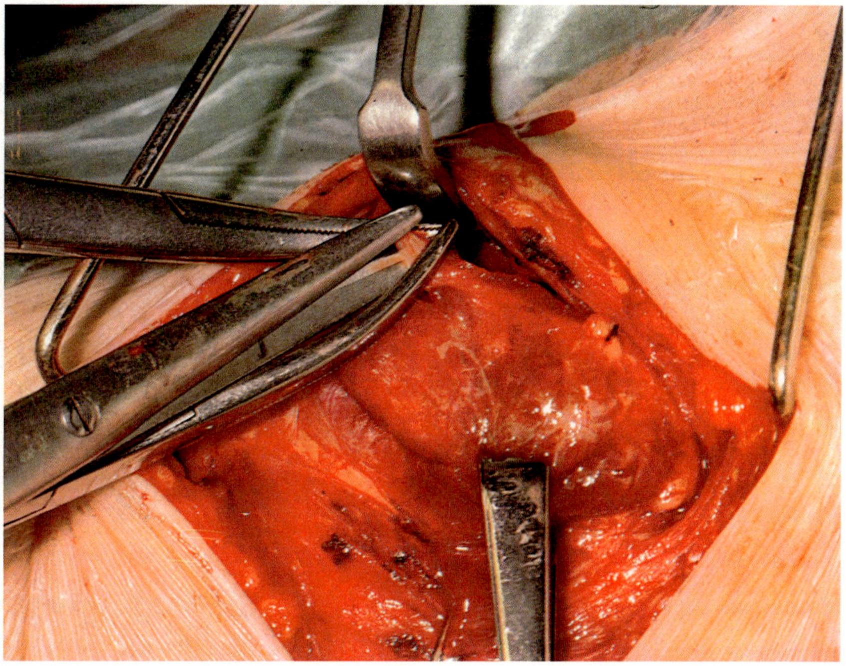

14 Inferior thyroid artery. The inferior thyroid artery, which can also vary in its position, is sought well away from the gland near to its point of emergence from deep to the common carotid artery. The inferior thyroid artery is here held up (but not secured) by artery forceps; the common carotid artery is the lighter coloured structure just beneath the upper retractor.

14

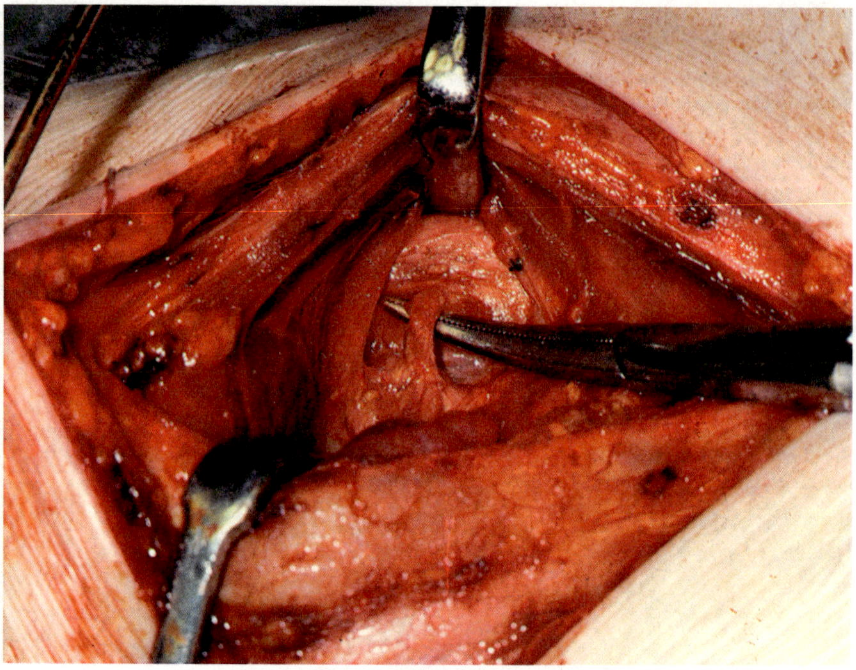

15 Temporary clamping of inferior thyroid artery. The inferior thyroid artery may be ligated in continuity or clamped temporarily by a bulldog clamp as shown here. Temporary clamping allows a normal blood supply to be restored to the parathyroid glands when the clamp is removed.

15

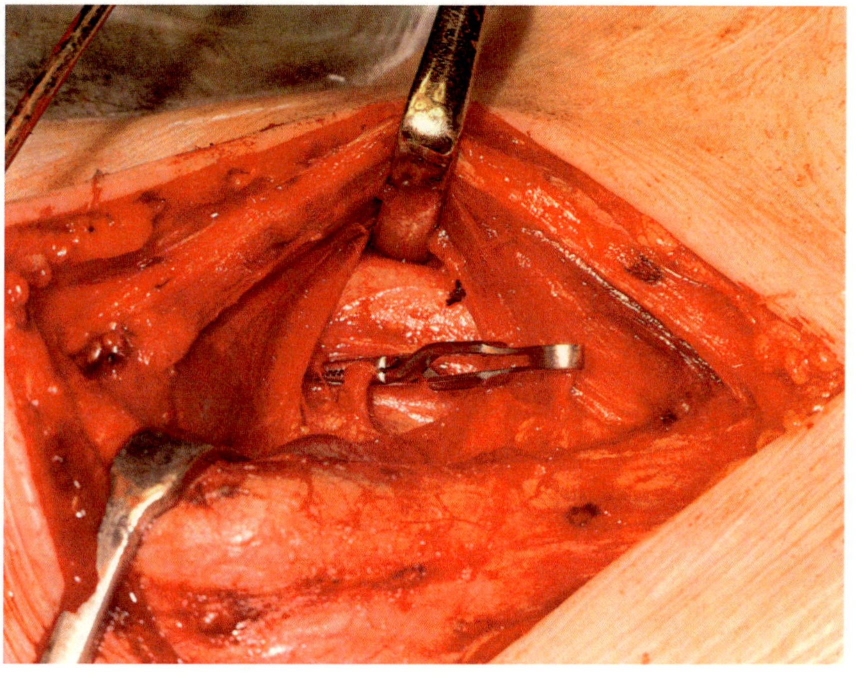

16 Upper pole exposed. The upper pole of the left thyroid lobe, containing the superior thyroid artery and vein, is now exposed. A finger is gently separating areolar tissue and the strap muscles away from the thyroid gland. The Dunhill double-hooked retractor under the strap muscles helps to provide a clearer view of the upper pole.

16

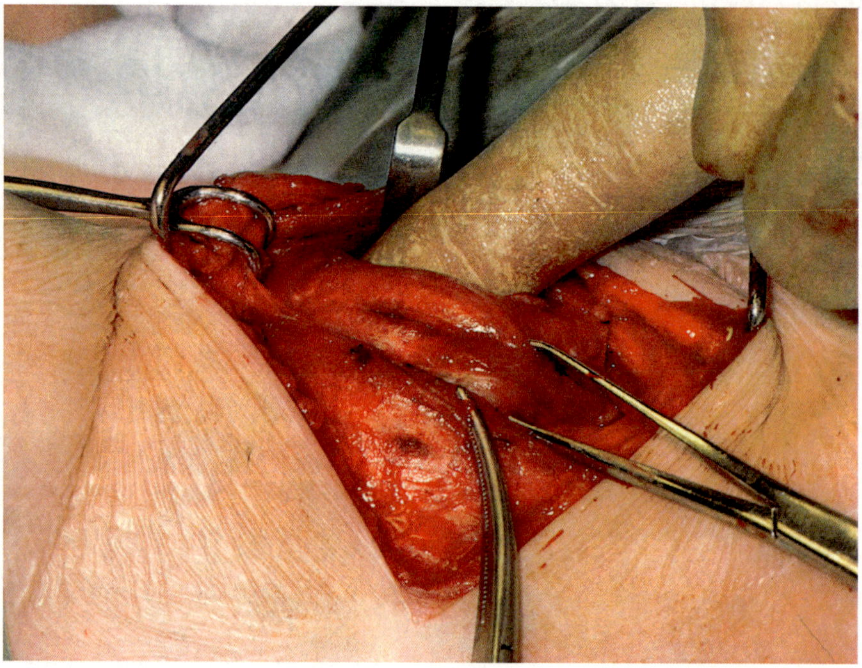

17 Scissor dissection of fascia. Fascia binding the upper pole to the trachea may need to be divided by scissor dissection before the upper pole can be fully mobilised preparatory to ligation and division of the superior thyroid vessels.

17

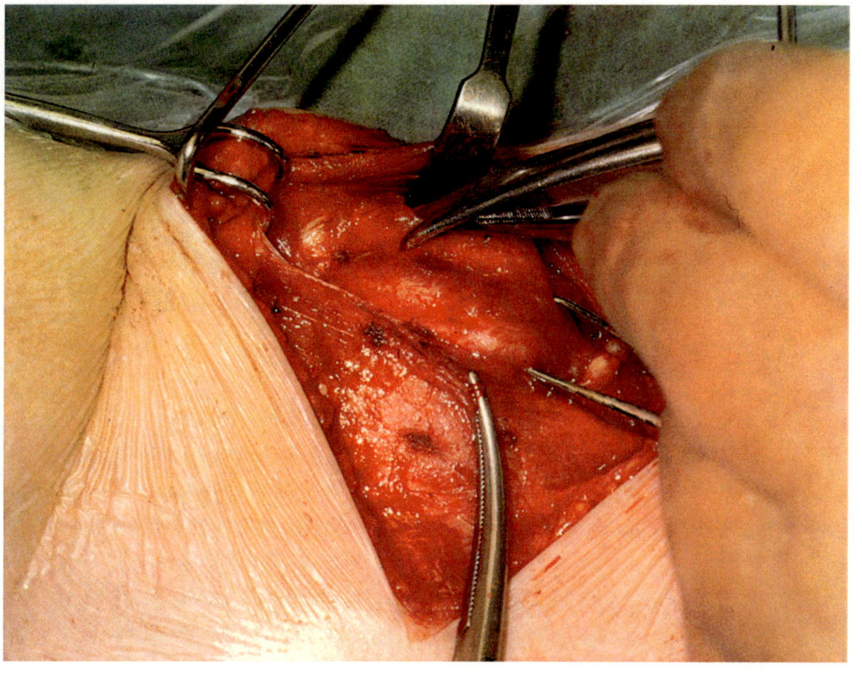

18 Upper pole grasped. The upper pole is being grasped between the operator's finger and thumb and drawn downwards.

18

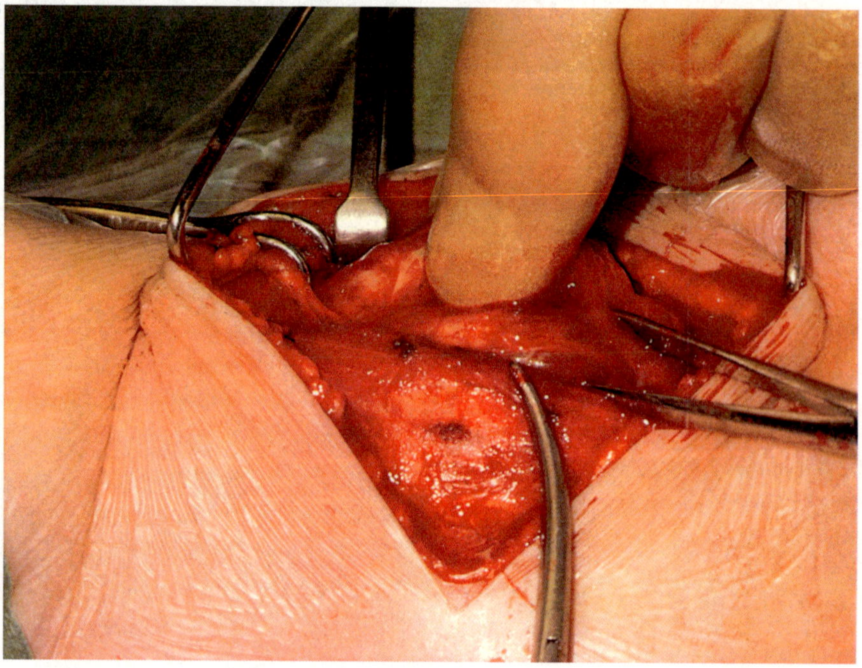

19 Use of thyroid dissector. A Kocher's thyroid dissector has been passed deep to the upper pole.

19

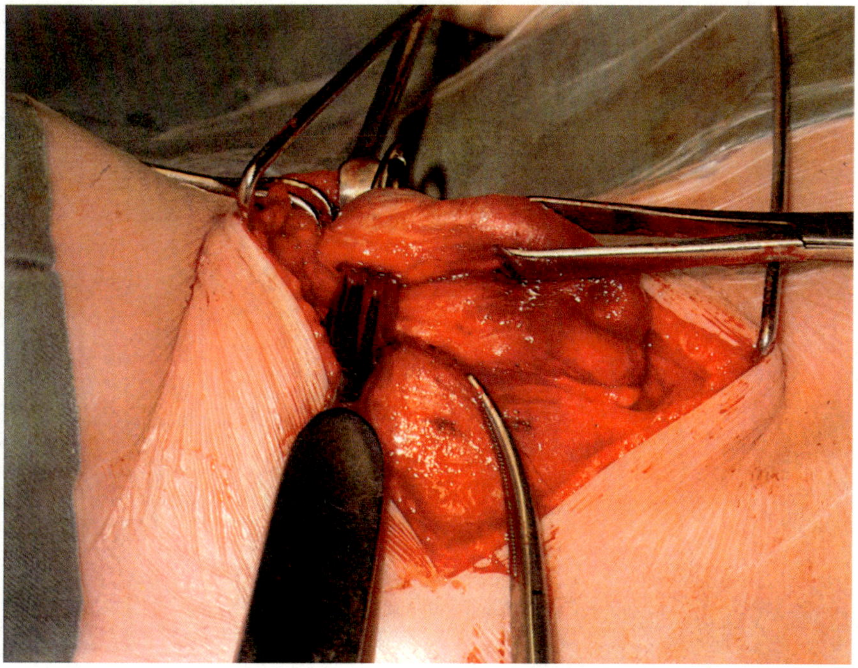

20 Dissection and clamping of upper pole. Three artery forceps are now placed across the upper pole vessels. The lowest artery forceps may include thyroid tissue. The dissection of the upper pole should be kept close to the thyroid gland so that the possibility of injury to the external laryngeal nerve is reduced; minor voice changes after operation can be caused by damage to this nerve.

20

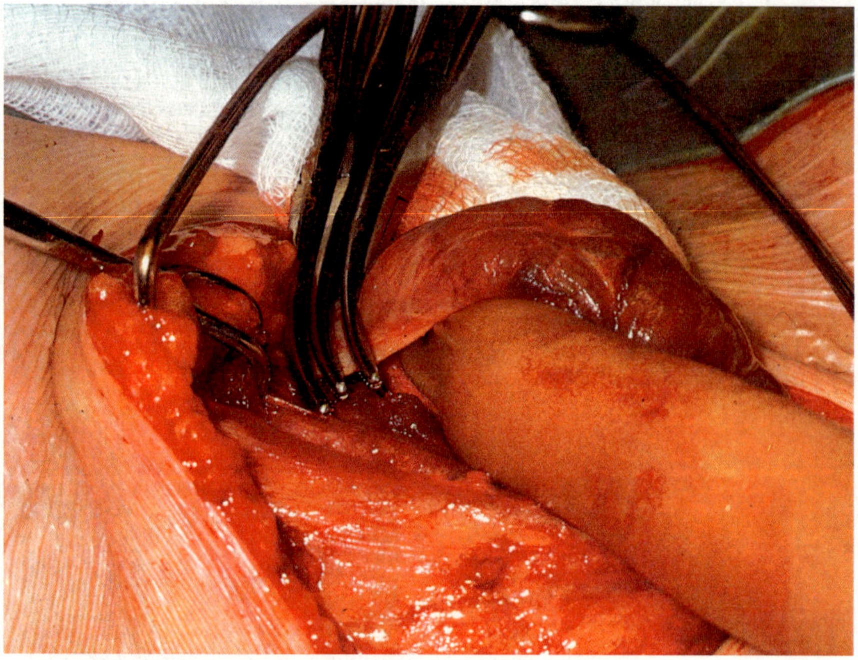

21 Division of vessels. The vessels are divided between the lower and upper two artery forceps. It is a wise precaution to place two artery forceps above, as the vessels can slip out of one pair of artery forceps and cause troublesome bleeding. If this does happen, finger pressure applied through the skin above the wound will control the bleeding and enable the cut ends of the vessels to be picked up.

21

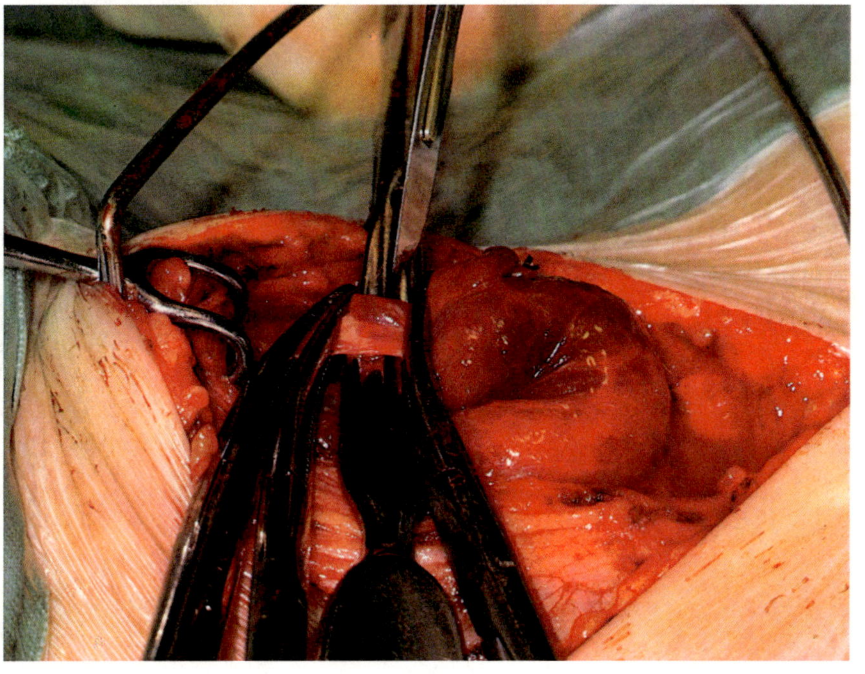

22 Applying ligatures. Two ligatures are applied to the proximal cut ends of the vessels. Here the second of the two ligatures is being tied. The distal cut ends of the vessels are then tied on the thyroid gland.

22

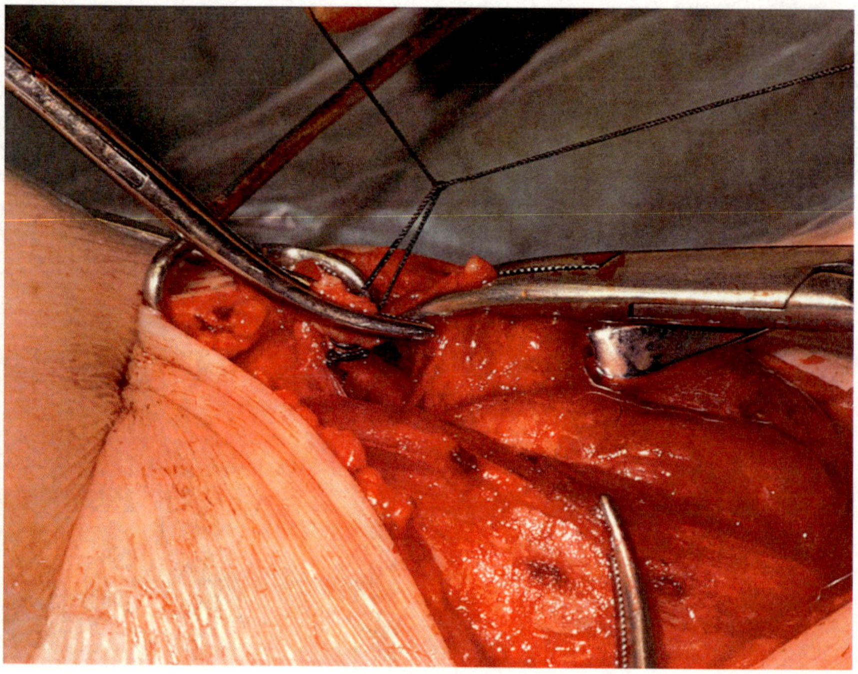

23 Posterolateral structures exposed. The left thyroid lobe is now pulled medially to expose the structures lying posterolaterally. The bull-dog clamp remains on the inferior thyroid artery; the dissecting forceps point to the recurrent laryngeal nerve lying in the groove between the trachea and the oesophagus. Note its relationship to the branching inferior thyroid artery. When not seen, the nerve may be identified by gently rolling it against the trachea, when it can be felt as a fine cord.

23

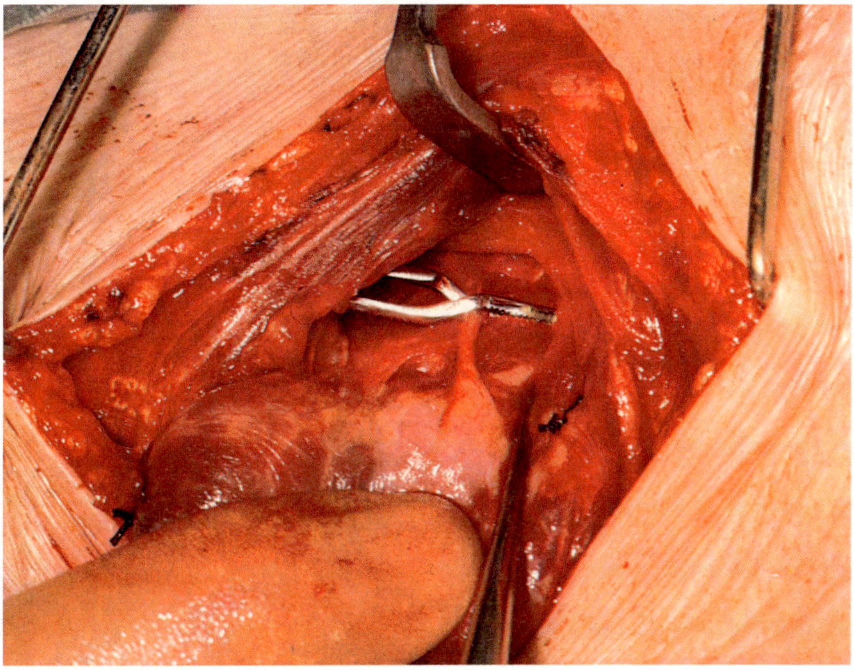

24 Parathyroid glands. The dissecting forceps point to the upper left parathyroid gland. The lower left parathyroid gland is lying deep to fascia just anterior to the recurrent laryngeal nerve, where the inferior thyroid artery is beginning to branch; it is difficult to identify in this photograph. No attempt is made to mobilise the parathyroid glands unless they lie on a part of the thyroid gland which is to be removed.

24

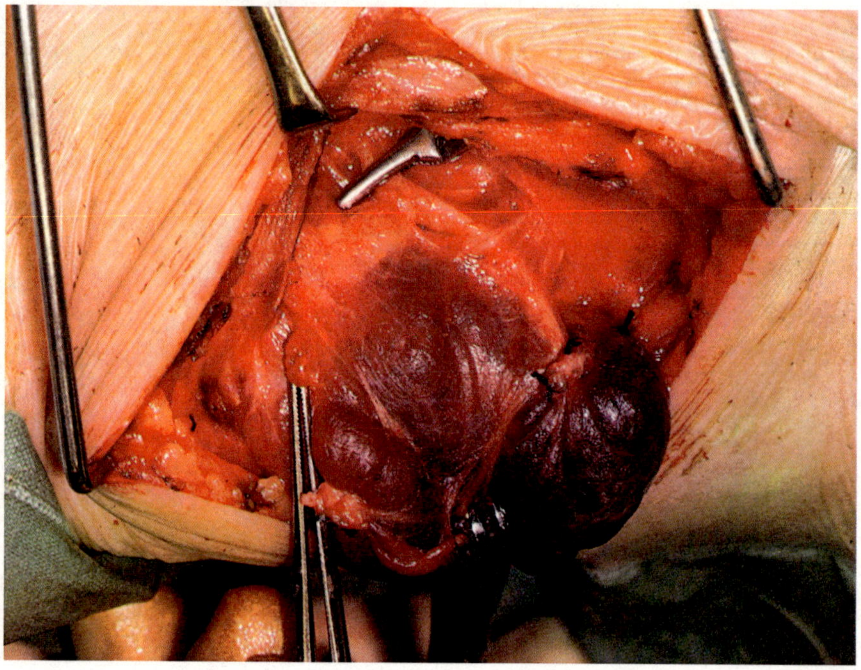

25 Inferior thyroid veins. The lower pole of the left thyroid lobe is now pulled upwards to demonstrate the inferior thyroid veins (the lower pole also contains fatty tissue, an occasional artery and, in some younger patients, the upper part of the thymus gland). Here some of the veins and fatty tissue are held in artery forceps ready for ligation. The main inferior thyroid veins are seen lying on the trachea deep to the artery forceps.

25

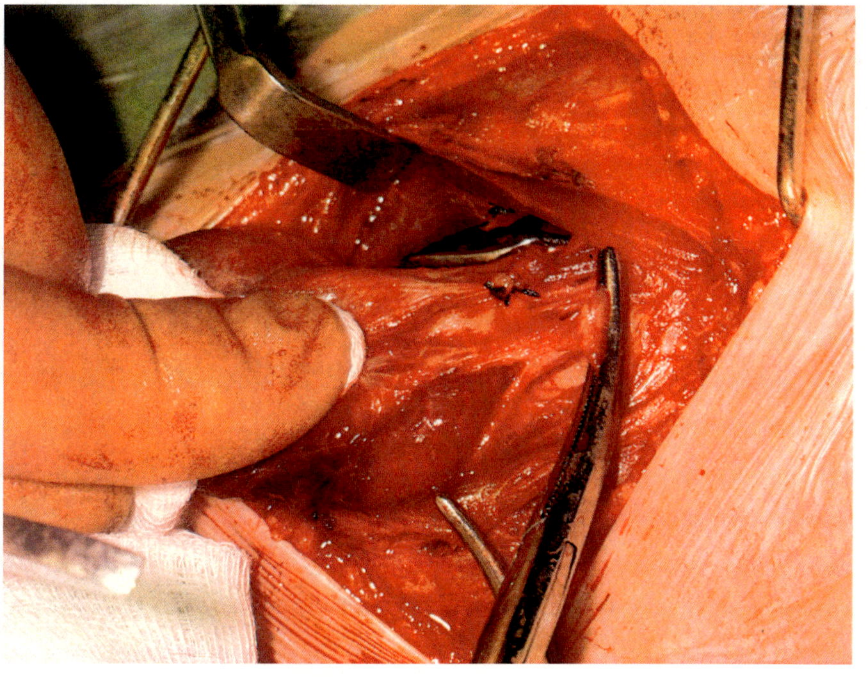

26 Divided and ligated lower pole vessels. The lower pole vessels have now been divided and ligated; two rings of the trachea can be seen at the tip of the Kocher's dissector.

26

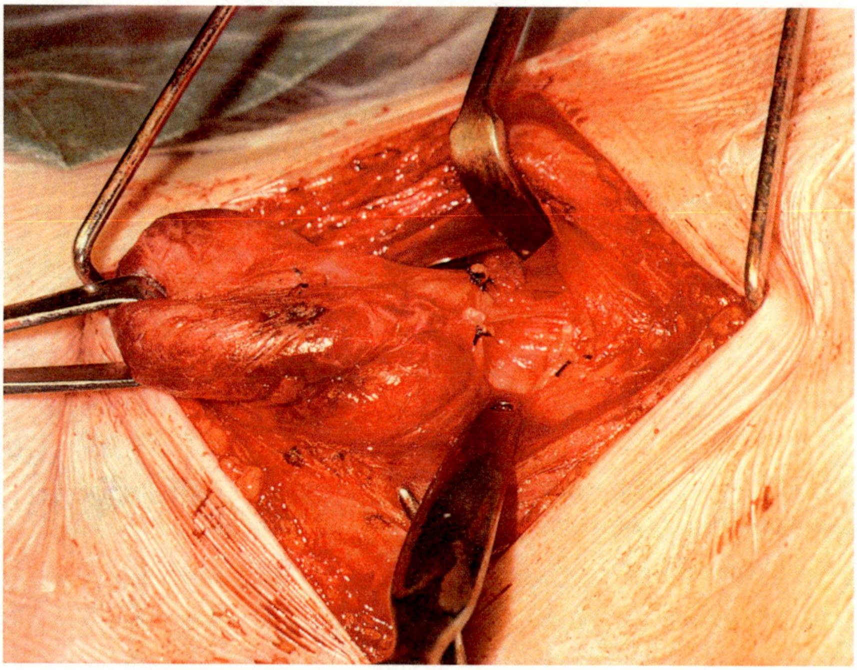

27 Trachea identification. The tip of the Kocher's dissector is now pointing to the trachea above the left thyroid lobe. It is obscured by the pyramidal lobe which will be removed later. The identification of the trachea above and below the left thyroid lobe is a necessary preliminary to the next step in the operation.

27

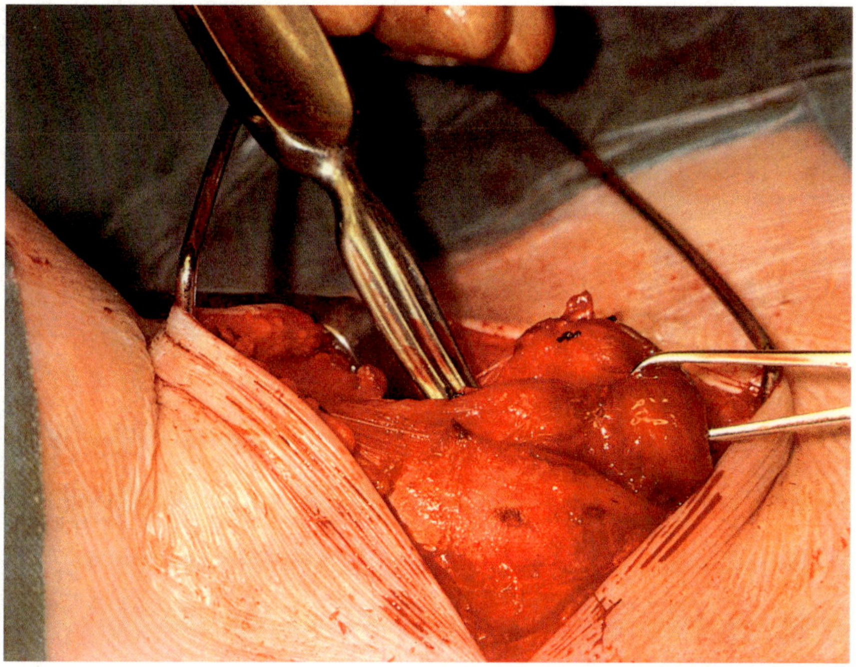

28 Kocher's dissector passed deep to thyroid isthmus. The Kocher's dissector is now passed deep to the isthmus of the thyroid gland and in front of the trachea as the left thyroid lobe is pulled forwards and medially. Artery forceps are to be applied to the thyroid capsule, but before this is done, the position of the parathyroid glands and the recurrent laryngeal nerve should be checked again.

28

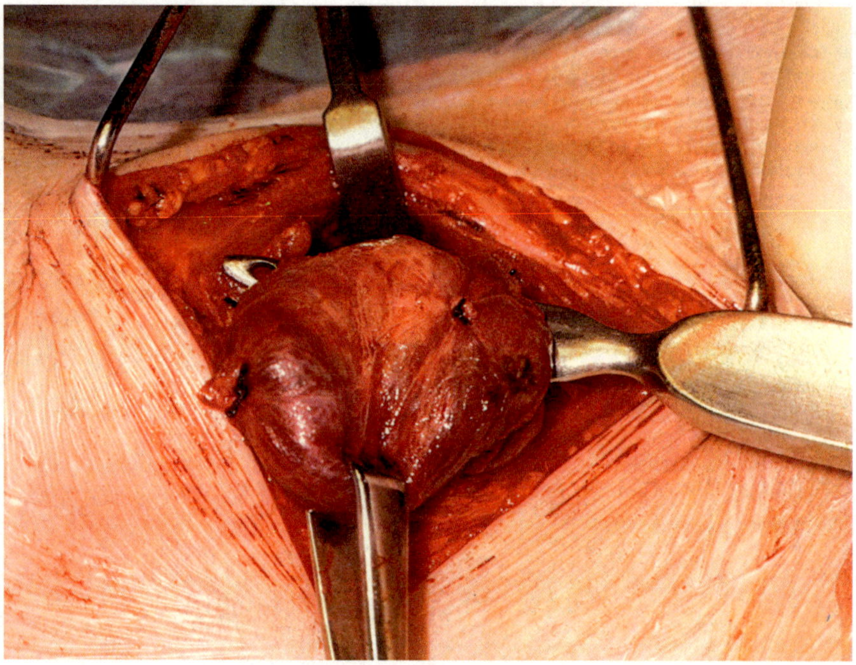

29 Checking position of parathyroid glands and recurrent laryngeal nerve. In this view, with the Kocher's dissector in position and the gland pulled medially, the relationship of the dissector to the recurrent laryngeal nerve and parathyroid glands is shown. The recurrent laryngeal nerve is seen crossing the inferior thyroid artery well behind the Kocher's dissector and the two parathyroid glands are in line with the lateral margin of the Kocher's dissector, so that artery forceps placed on the thyroid capsule just anterior to the guide will avoid injury to these structures.

29

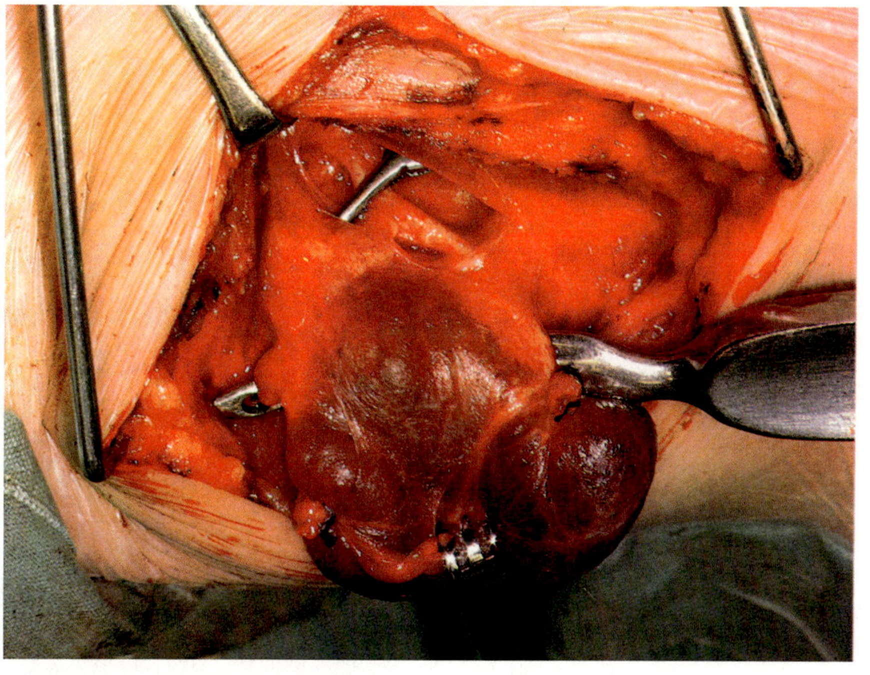

Excision of left thyroid lobe

30 Positioning of artery forceps on posterolateral capsule. A row of artery forceps are now placed on the capsule of the posterolateral part of the thyroid lobe, their precise positioning will depend upon how much of the thyroid lobe is to be removed. Division of the thyroid lobe by knife dissection can now begin.

30

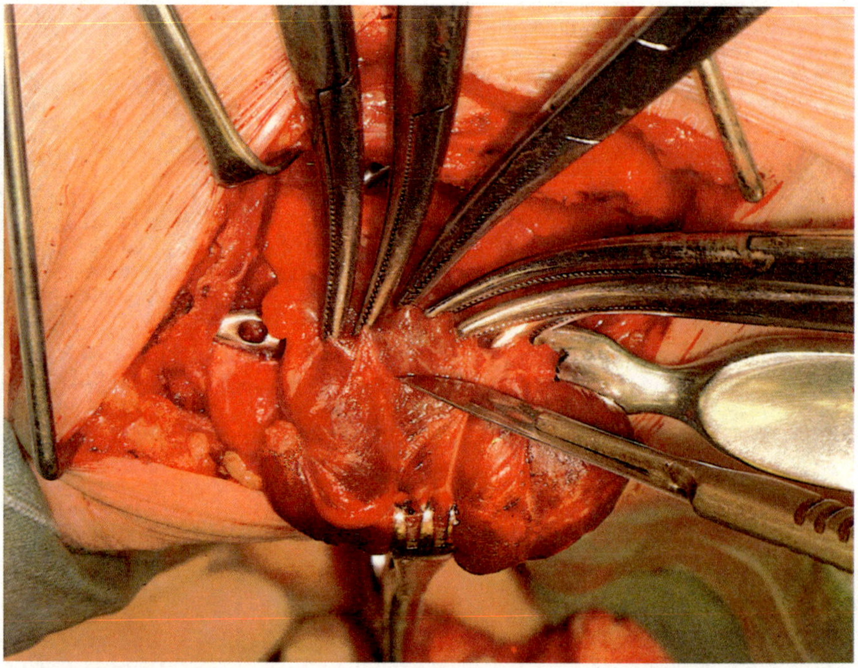

31 Knife dissection of left lobe and control of bleeding points. Most of the bleeding points are in or near the thyroid capsule and are controlled by the artery forceps which have been already placed. Bleeding points within the substance of the gland are picked up by artery forceps and ligated or coagulated as the dissection proceeds.

31

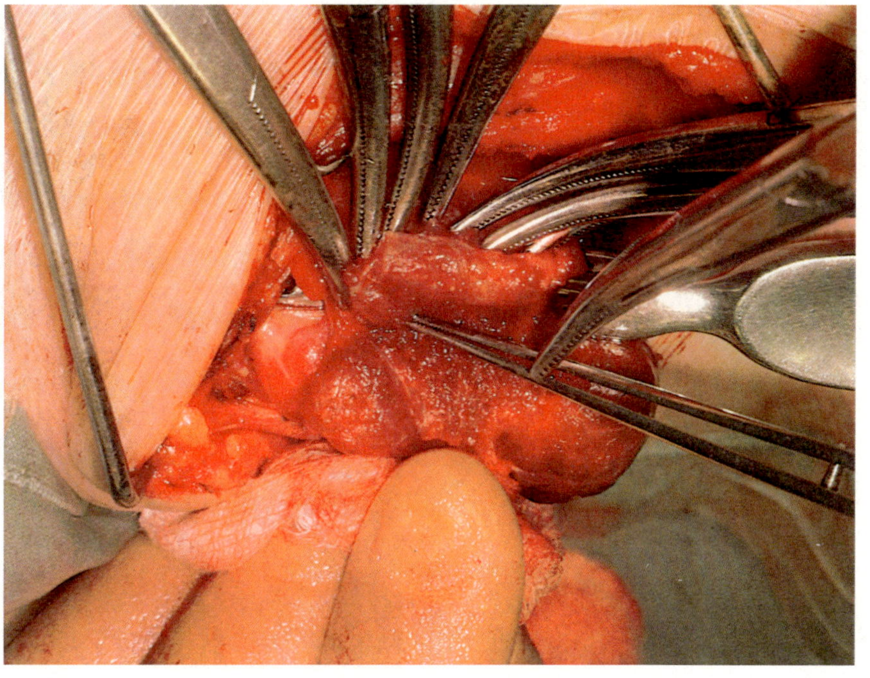

32 Artery forceps on posteromedial capsule. When the capsule of the posteromedial part of the thyroid lobe is reached, it is picked up in a series of artery forceps in a similar manner to those placed on the posterolateral thyroid capsule. Here the posteromedial capsule is being divided; when division is complete, the Kocher's dissector is removed.

32

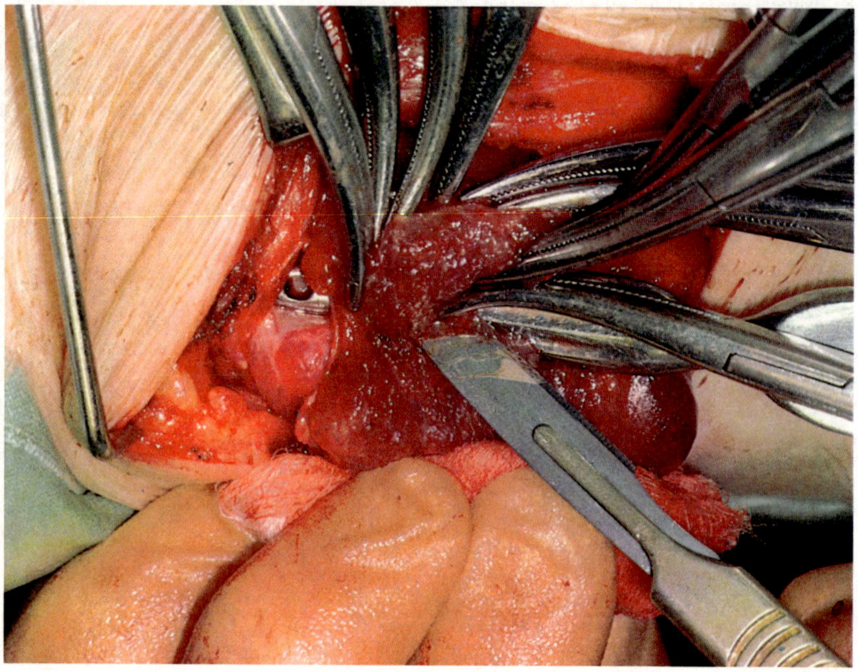

33 Subtotal removal of left thyroid lobe is complete with artery forceps in position, awaiting ligature. All the artery forceps are in position. The posteromedial capsule has been divided. Ligatures are now applied around each artery forceps in turn.

33

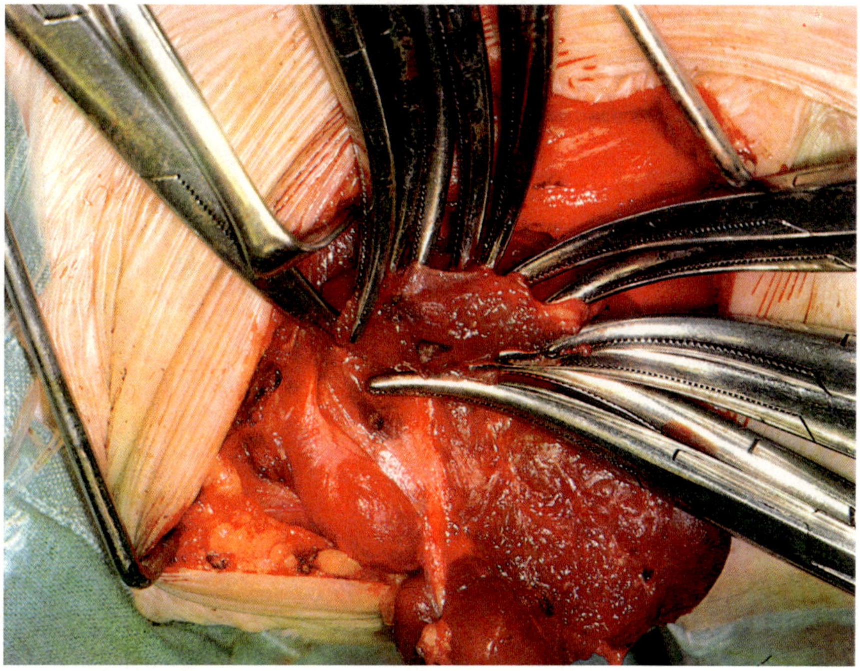

34 Fixation of left lobe remnant. The remnant of the left thyroid lobe, free from bleeding, is now ready to be stitched to the side of the trachea by several interrupted sutures of 2/0 chromic catgut placed between the posterolateral thyroid capsule and the connective tissue covering the side of the trachea. The first of these sutures is being tied.

34

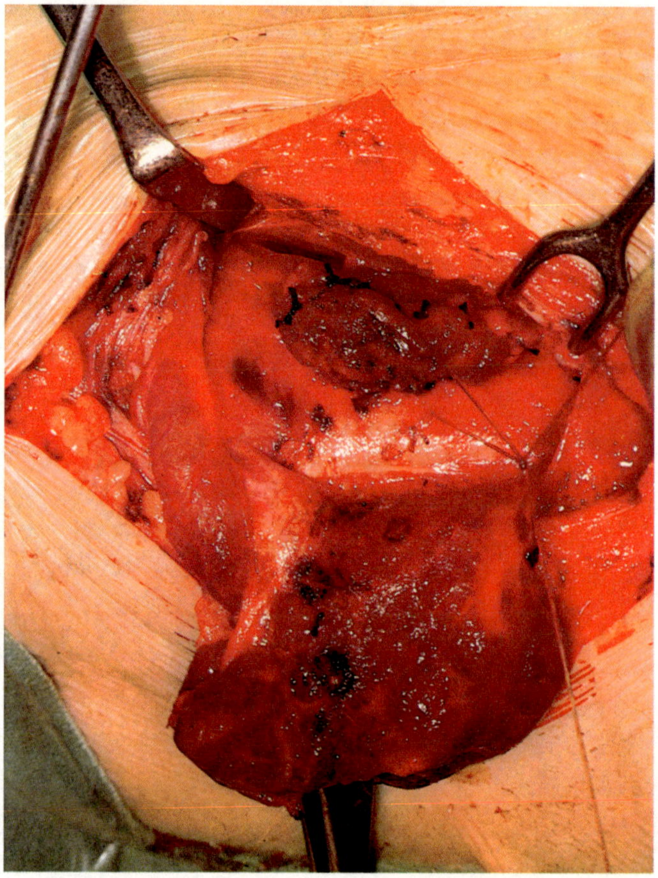

35 Care of laryngeal nerve and parathyroid glands. With the catgut sutures tied, the left thyroid lobe remnant lies snugly against the side of the trachea; any oozing from the cut surface is thus controlled. Care must be taken to avoid including the recurrent laryngeal nerve and the parathyroid glands in these sutures. The bulldog clamp can now be removed from the inferior thyroid artery.

35

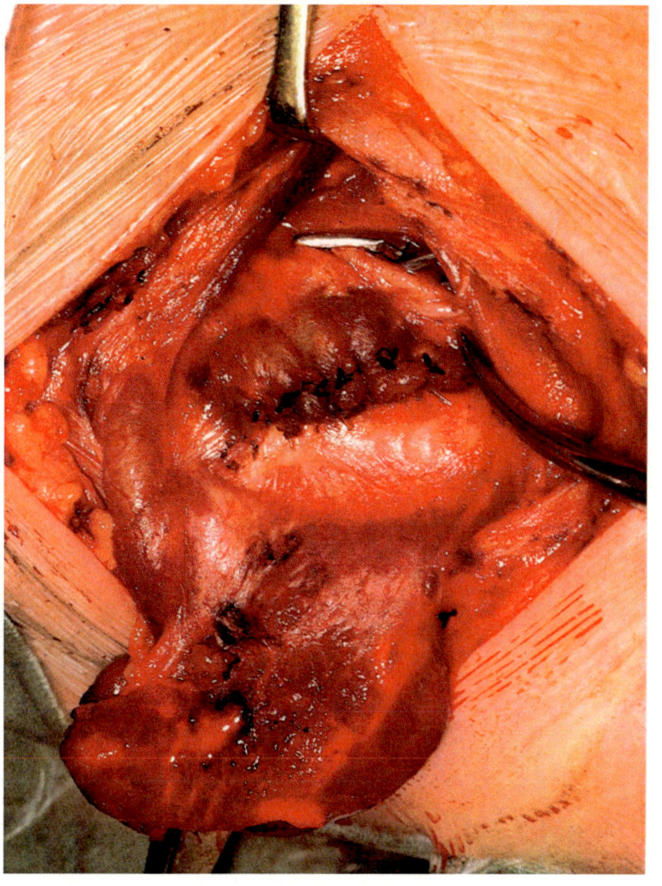

Excision of pyramidal lobe and thyroid isthmus

36 Dissection of pyramidal lobe. When a pyramidal lobe is present it should be dissected free and removed with the main specimen. It is shown being lifted up by artery forceps. It has a rich blood supply and several vessels have usually to be ligated and divided, before it is freed.

36

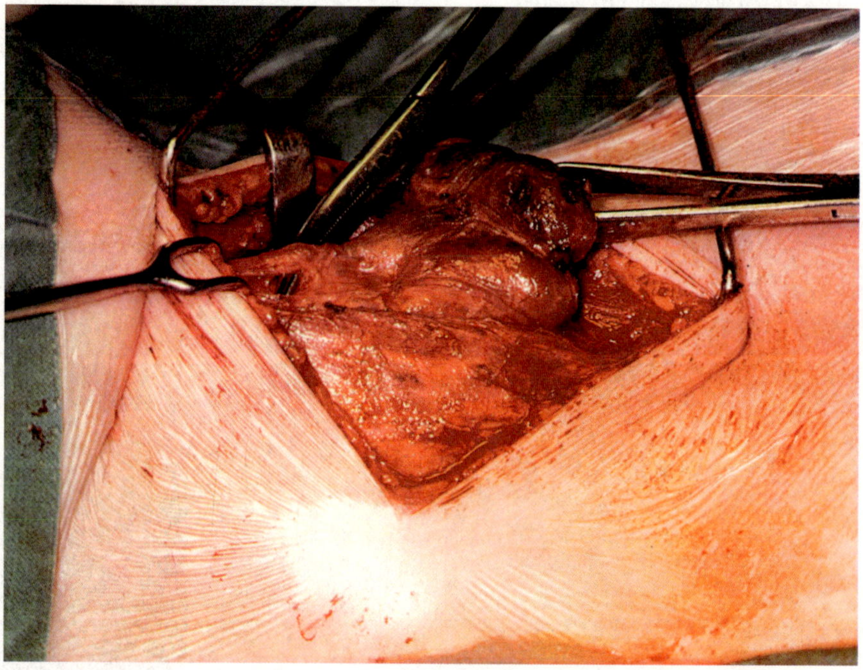

37 Excision of pyramidal lobe and isthmus. Finally, the upper extremity of the pyramidal lobe is divided between two artery forceps. Both cut ends are ligated. This completes the left side of the operation. The pyramidal lobe remains attached to the thyroid isthmus, which is lifted off the trachea by blunt or sharp dissection.

37

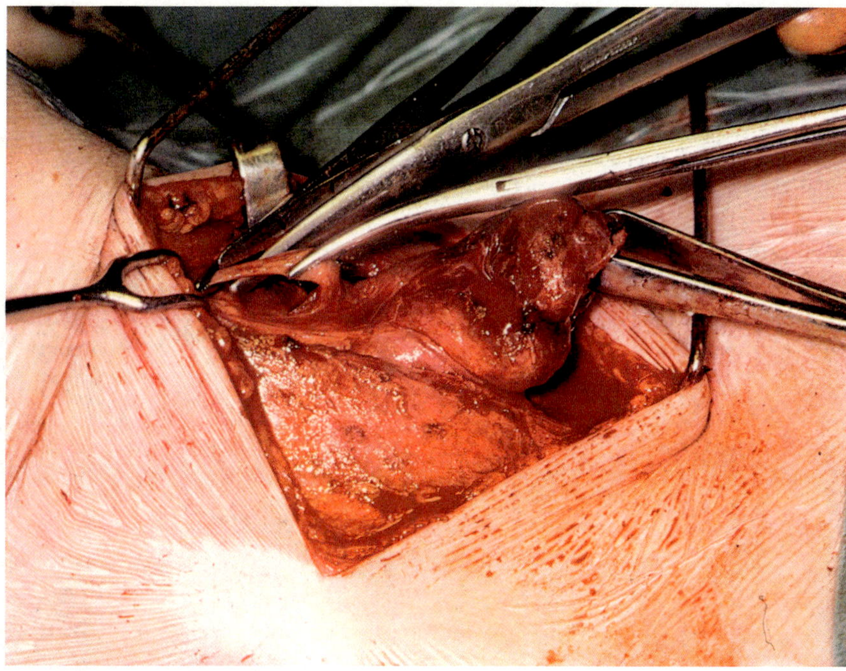

Mobilisation of right thyroid lobe

38 Right strap muscles retraction. The surgeon is now standing on the left side of the patient for the next stage of the operation, which is mobilisation of the right thyroid lobe. The strap muscles are being retracted and separated from the underlying thyroid lobe. This may be done by finger or scissor dissection depending upon the consistency of this tissue, which varies from individual to individual.

38

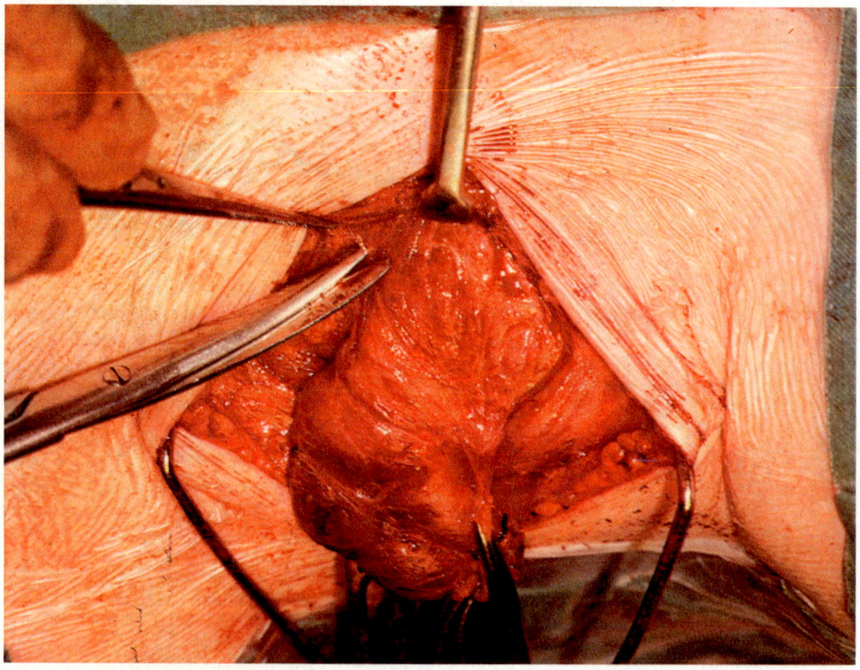

39 Middle thyroid vein. The middle thyroid vein is seen running across the common carotid artery from the posterolateral part of the thyroid gland. It will be divided between ligatures to provide access to the side and back of the right thyroid lobe.

39

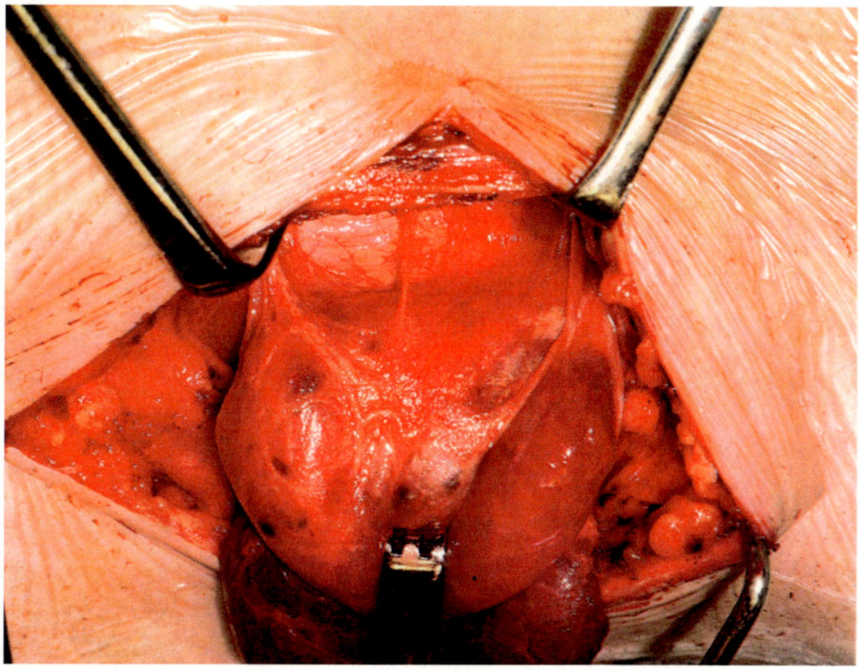

40 Inferior thyroid artery. The inferior thyroid artery is mobilised as it emerges from deep to the common carotid artery. It will be occluded temporarily with a bulldog clamp. The recurrent laryngeal nerve is seen crossing the inferior thyroid artery nearer to the thyroid gland.

40

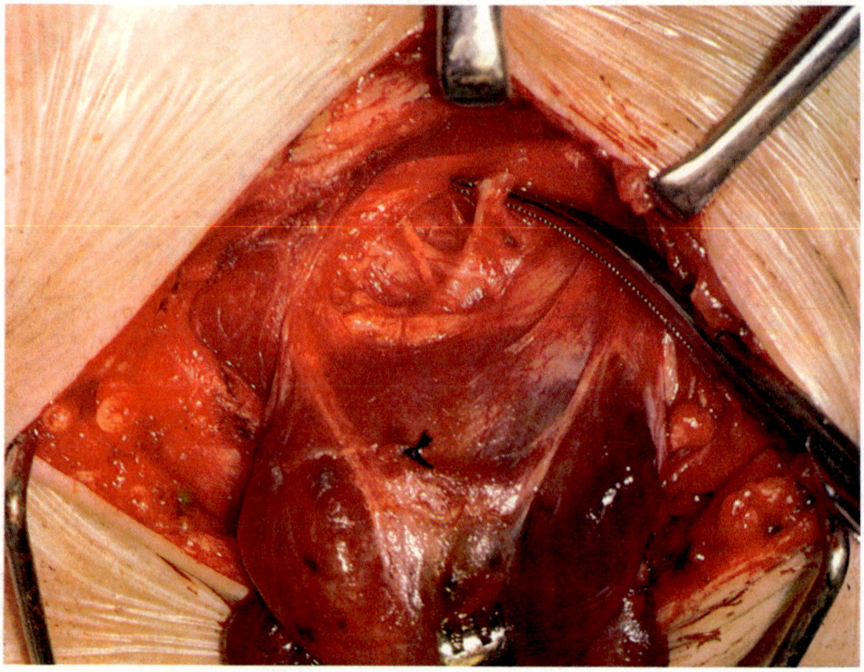

41 Mobilisation of right upper pole. The right upper pole is now mobilised and a Kocher's dissector passed deep to it. The upper pole generally extends higher on the right than on the left side and a tongue of thyroid gland often passes medially deep to the pharynx. This may make mobilisation of the right upper pole a little more difficult than on the left side. This 'tongue' is not clearly shown here but it can be seen on the operation specimen (**58**).

41

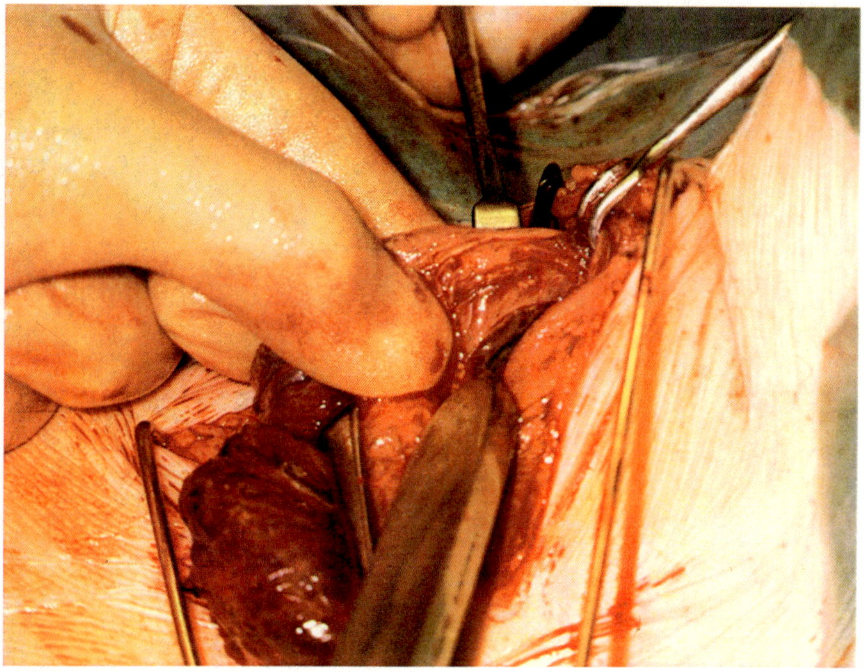

42 Superior thyroid artery. In some instances it may be more expedient to take the upper pole vessels in two 'bites' rather than in a single manoeuvre. Here the superior thyroid artery is secured between two artery forceps and divided as it lies on the upper pole.

42

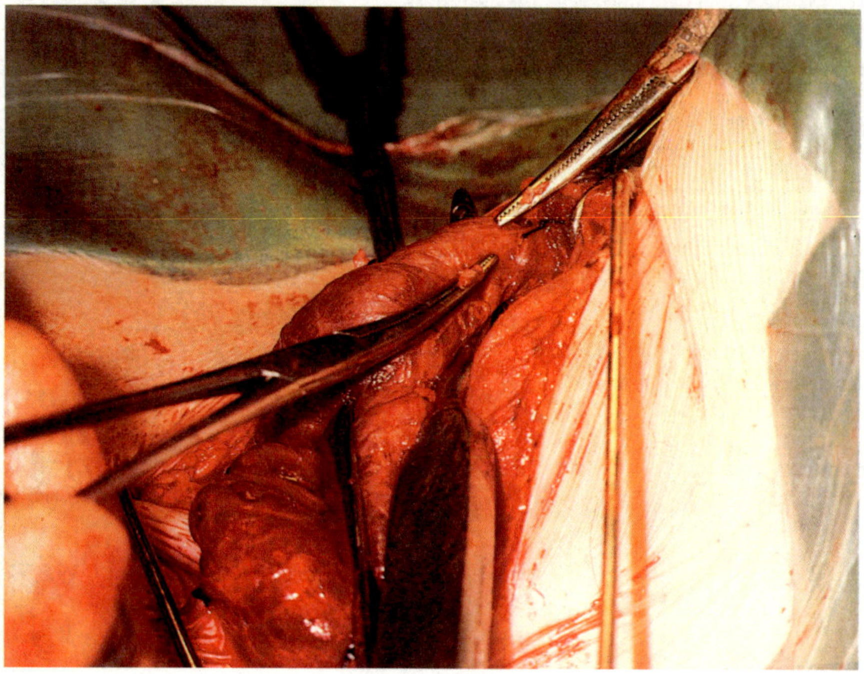

43 Remaining upper pole vessels secured. The remaining upper pole vessels have been secured in three artery forceps and are being divided by scissors between the lower and upper two artery forceps. Ligatures are then applied.

43

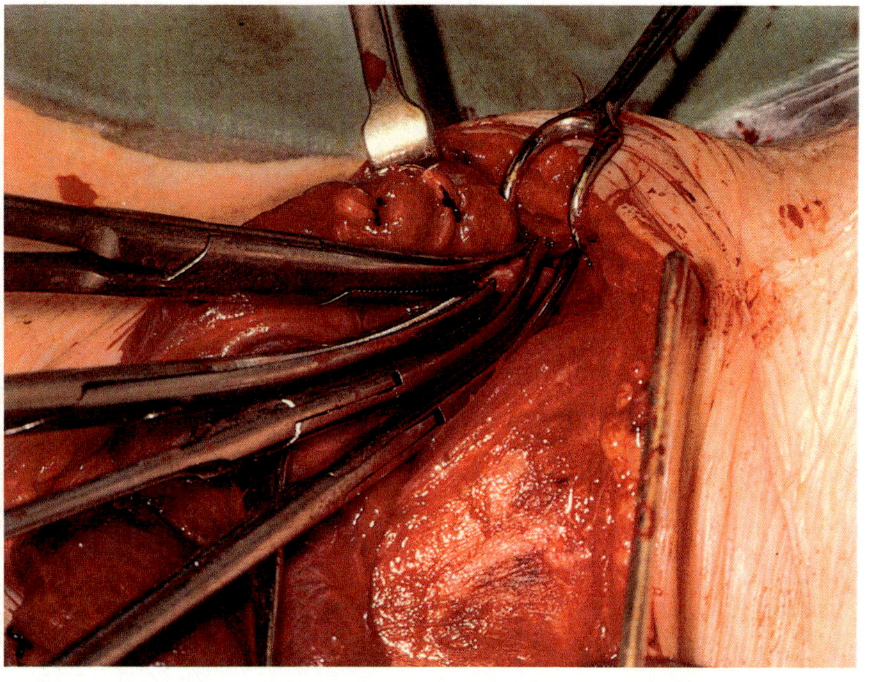

44 Inferior thyroid veins. This view is taken from below the wound and shows the right thyroid lobe being drawn upwards. The leash of inferior thyroid veins lie between the tip of the artery forceps and the retractor. They are secured in two artery forceps, divided and ligated.

44

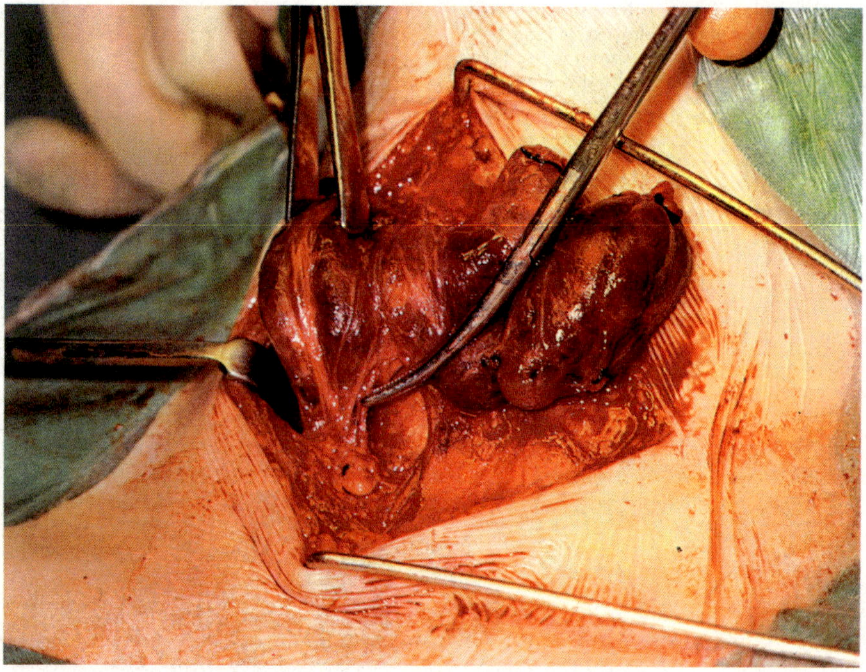

45 Posteromedial aspect of lobe exposed. The right thyroid lobe is being lifted forwards and laterally to expose the posteromedial aspect of the lobe where it is attached to the side of the trachea by fairly dense fascia. This fascia is being divided by the scalpel. This dissection must be limited to a depth of 1mm or 2mm only. Small vessels are secured on the capsule of the thyroid gland with artery forceps. If this dissection is made too deeply, troublesome bleeding may occur and the recurrent nerve will be in danger of injury, particularly in the upper more anterior part of its course just before it enters the larynx, behind the inferior cornu of the thyroid cartilage.

45

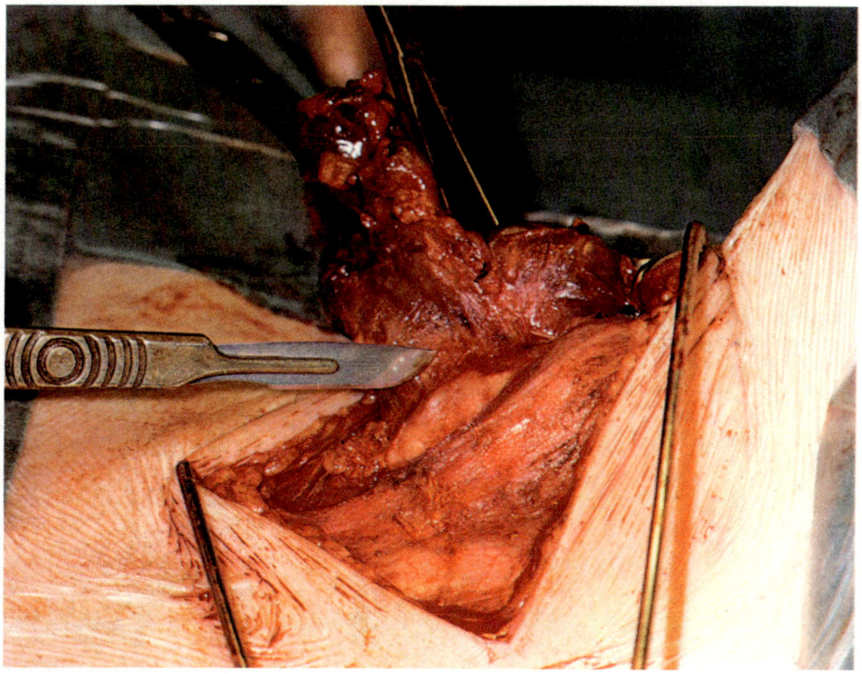

46 Posterolateral structures exposed. The right thyroid lobe is now pulled forwards and medially. Before placing a row of artery forceps on the posterolateral capsule of the thyroid lobe, preparatory to dividing it, an attempt should be made to locate the recurrent laryngeal nerve and the parathyroid glands.

The bulldog clamp is on the inferior thyroid artery; the tip of the dissecting forceps is pointing to the recurrent laryngeal nerve, which is running obliquely forwards to enter the larynx.

The parathyroid glands have not been clearly identified; however, so long as it can be seen that they are not lying on that part of the thyroid lobe which is to be removed, it is safe to proceed.

46

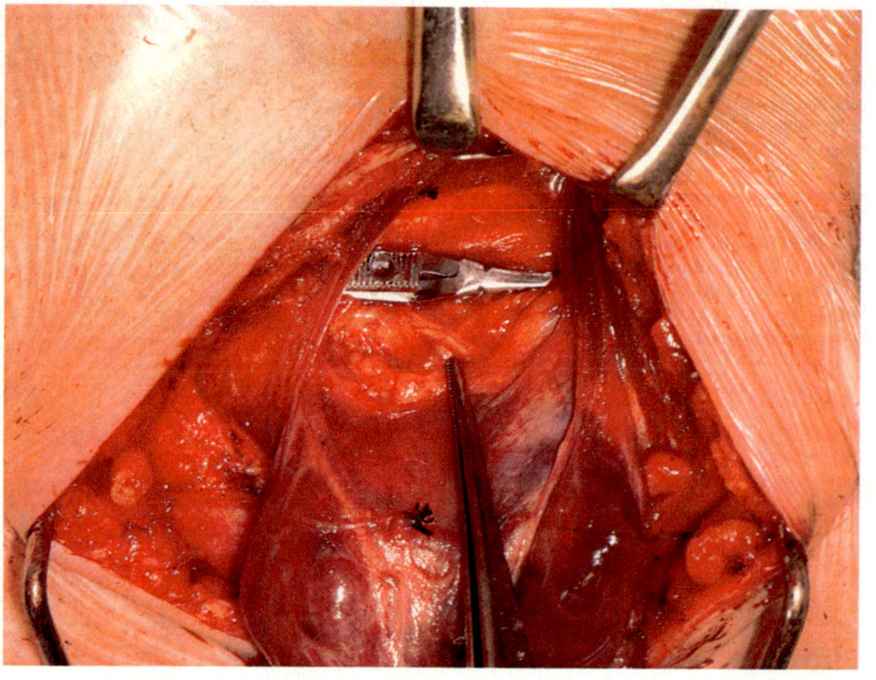

Excision of right thyroid lobe

47 Artery forceps on posterolateral thyroid capsule. A row of artery forceps are placed along the posterolateral thyroid capsule.

47

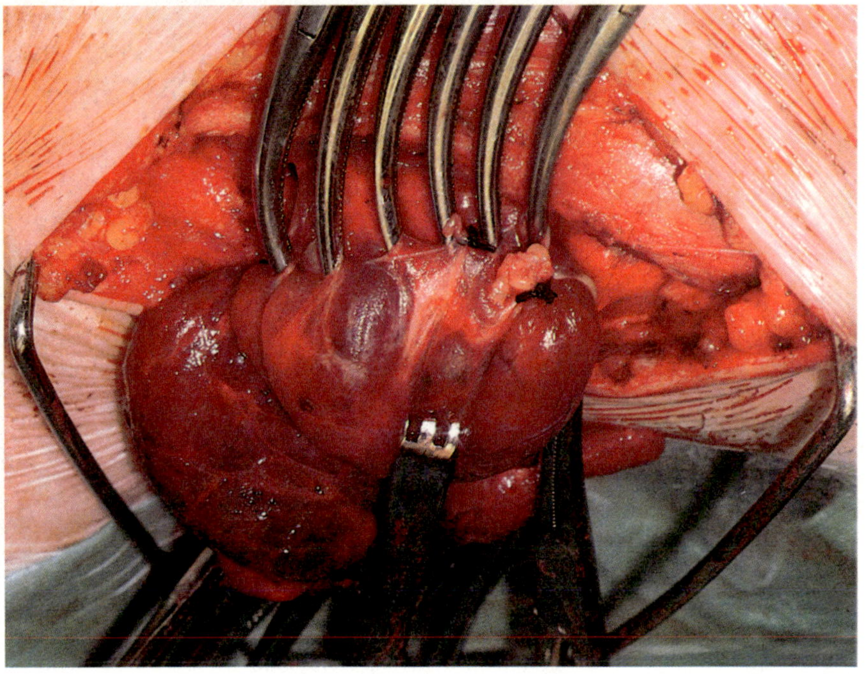

48 Artery forceps on posteromedial thyroid capsule. Similarly, a row of artery forceps are placed along the posteromedial thyroid capsule. Note that the posterior part of the lobe is still adherent to the trachea. The recurrent laryngeal nerve is not in danger, so long as the artery forceps are placed on the thyroid capsule and not on the trachea.

48

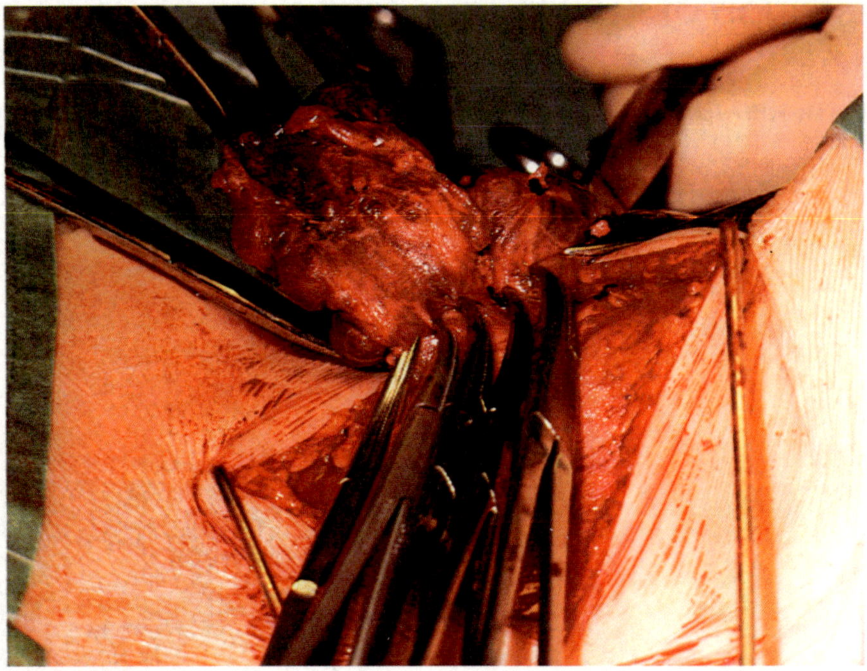

49 Knife dissection of right lobe. The desired amount of thyroid tissue is now removed by scalpel dissection. Bleeding points within the thyroid substance are picked up in artery forceps for ligation or coagulation. The dissection proceeds as far as the posteromedial thyroid capsule.

49

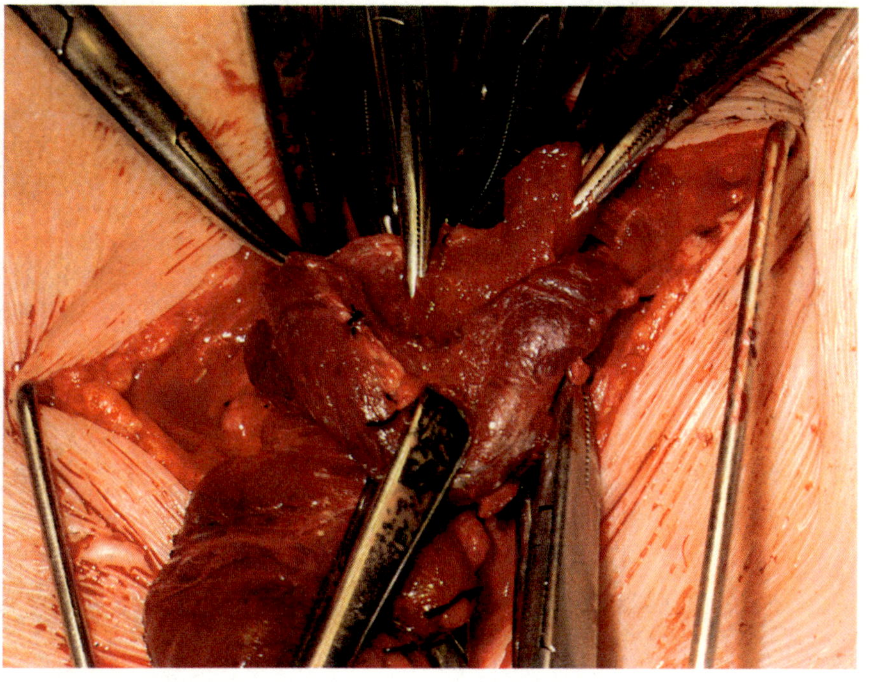

50 Subtotal removal of right thyroid lobe. With the thyroid gland pulled laterally, the posteromedial thyroid capsule is finally divided to complete the subtotal removal of the right thyroid lobe.

50

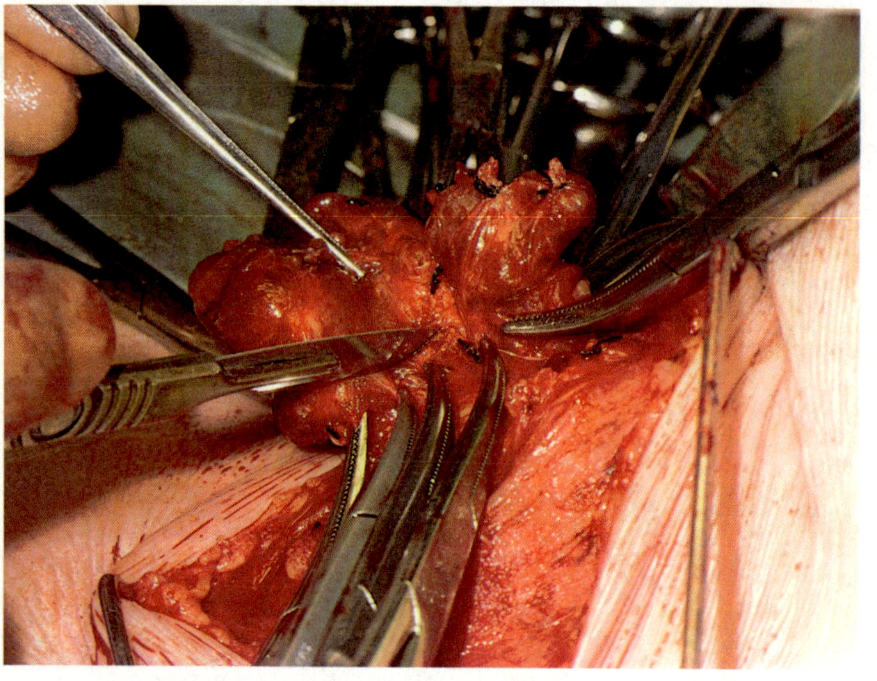

51 Artery forceps on bleeding points. Removal of the desired amount of the right thyroid lobe is complete and the remnant is seen with the artery forceps still in position awaiting ligation of the vessels within them.

51

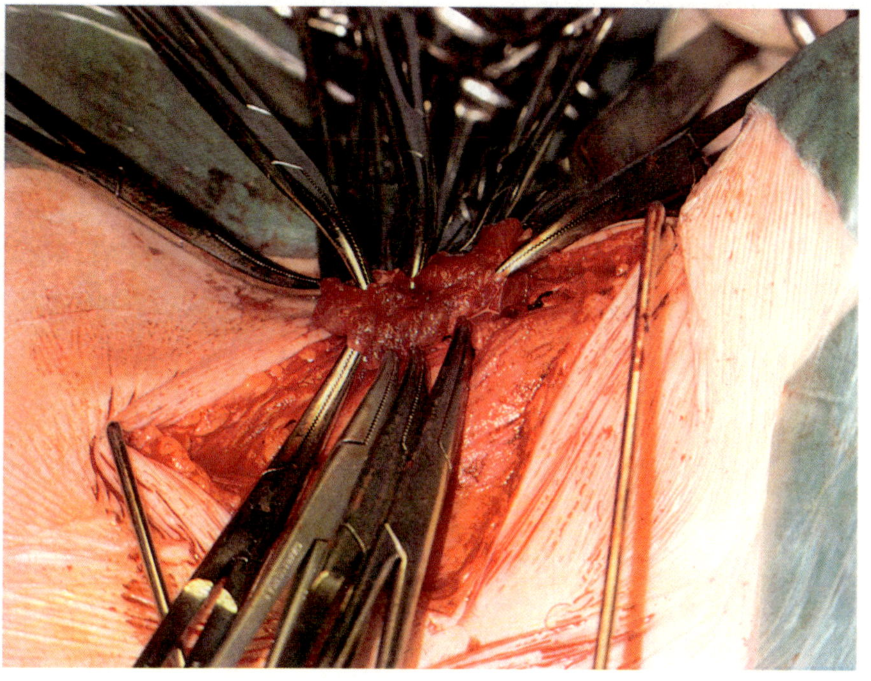

52 Remnant of right lobe awaiting fixation to trachea. The vessels have been ligated; the remnant is free from bleeding and is ready to be sutured to the side of the trachea with interrupted sutures of 2/0 chromic catgut.

52

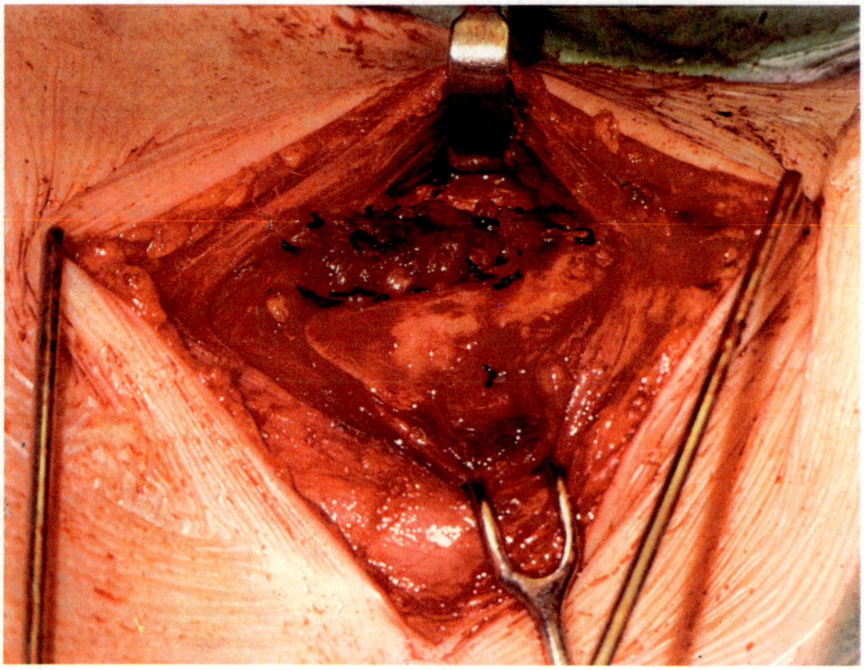

53 Both lobe remnants sutured to trachea. In this view, taken from below the wound, both thyroid lobe remnants are shown sutured to the sides of the trachea. Check that the bulldog clamps have been removed from each inferior thyroid artery.

53

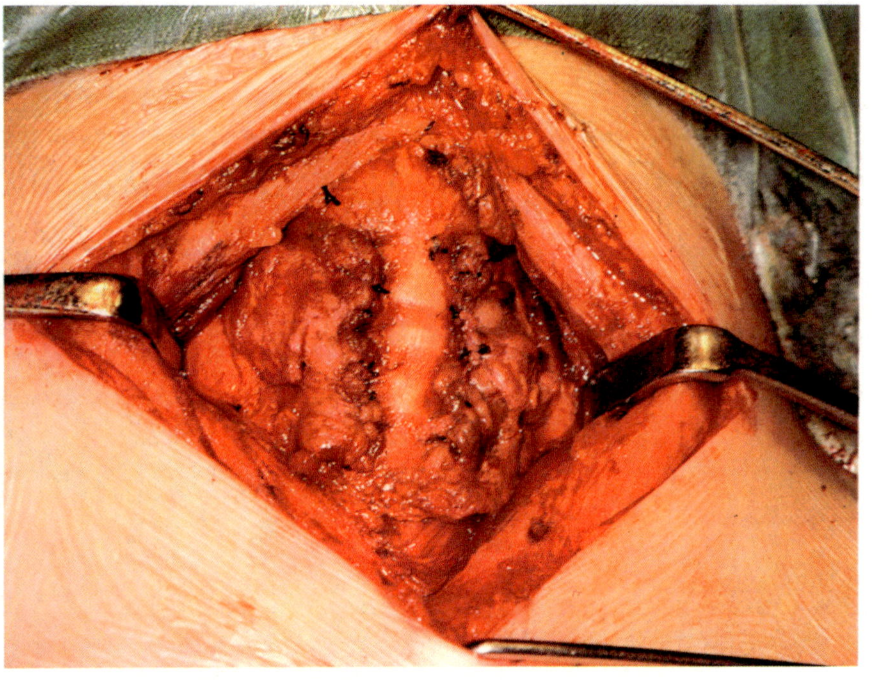

Suction drainage and wound closure

54 Suction drain placement. A Redivac suction drain is placed adjacent to each thyroid lobe remnant and brought through the muscles and the skin below the edge of the wound on the opposite side. Each drainage tube is attached to a separate suction bottle.

54

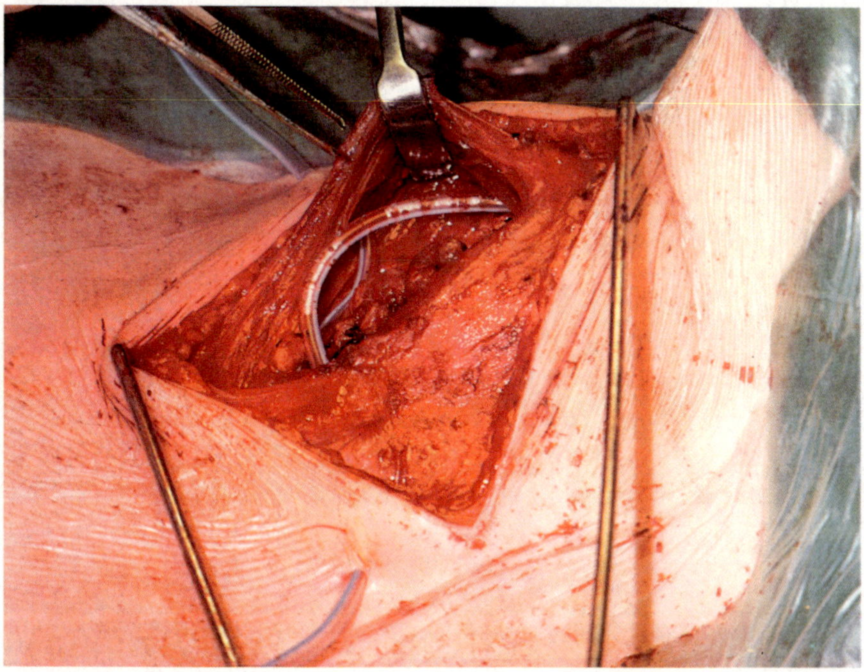

55 Approximation of strap muscles. The strap muscles are approximated in the midline by a continuous suture of 2/0 catgut placed through the fascia covering the muscles. Care must be taken to avoid the anterior jugular veins.

55

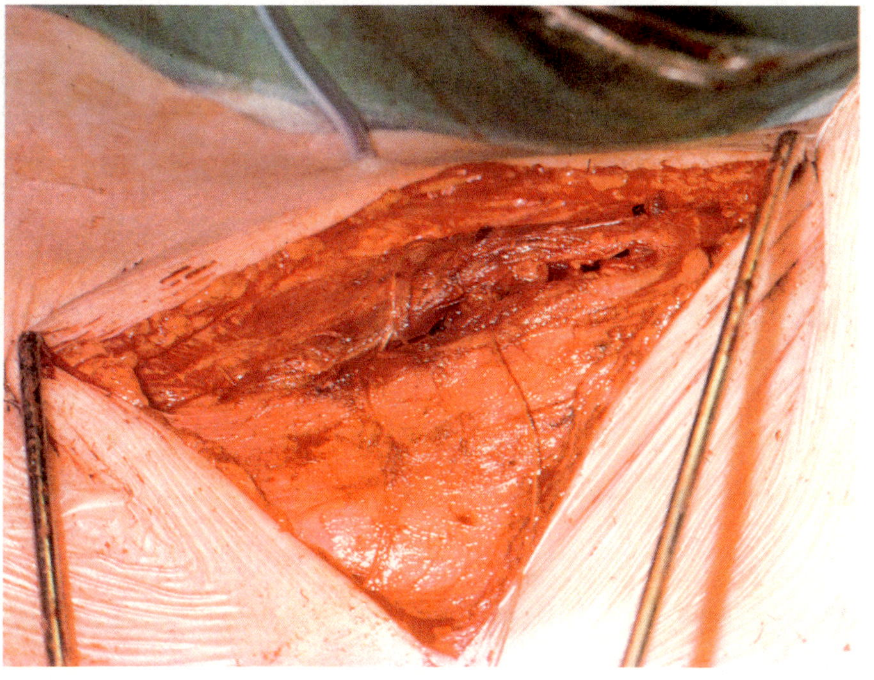

56 Control of bleeding points. Remaining bleeding points in the subcutaneous tissues are ligated or coagulated before the skin is closed. A separate suture for the platysma muscle is not necessary.

56

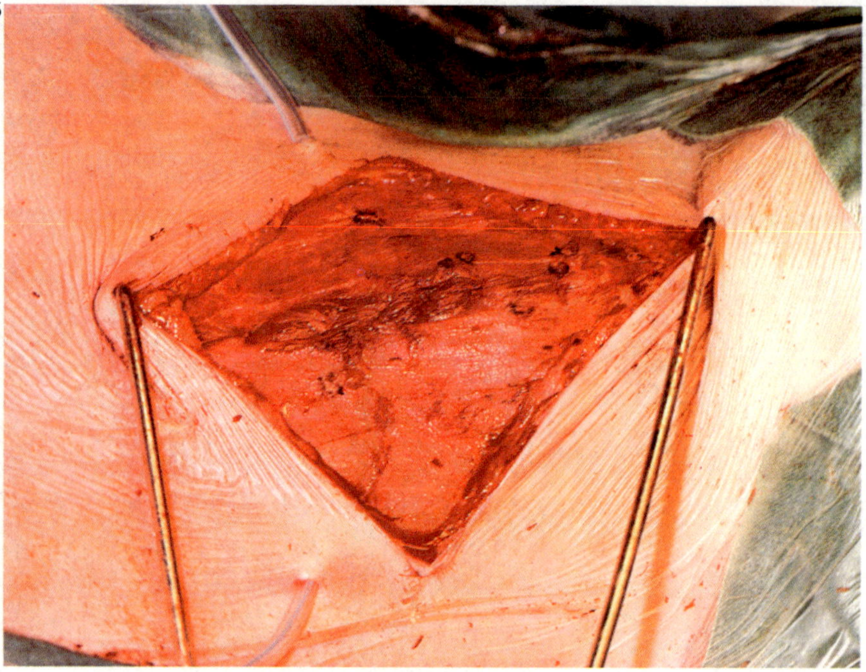

57

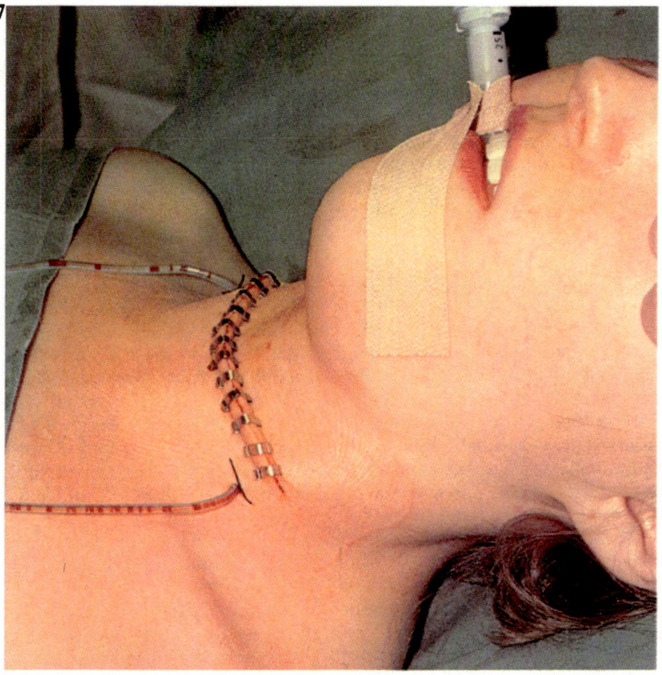

58

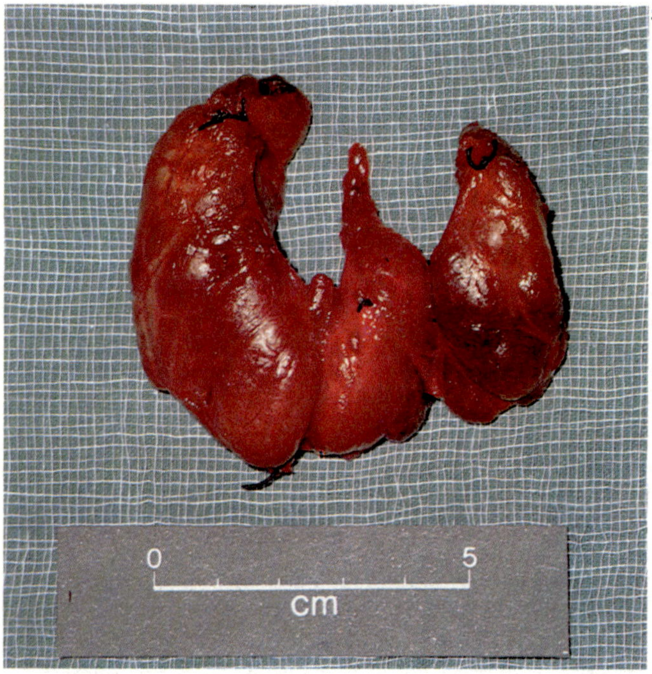

57 Approximation of skin edges. The skin edges are approximated with metal clips or sutures.

58 Operation specimen. The operation specimen shows both thyroid lobes joined by the isthmus and the pyramidal lobe. The higher right upper pole with its 'tongue' which lay behind the pharynx is clearly seen.

Postoperative management

Postoperative recovery is usually straightforward after thyroidectomy. The suction drains are removed along with half of the skin clips or sutures on the second postoperative day. The remaining skin clips are removed on the third postoperative day. The patient is discharged home on the fourth or fifth day after operation.

Early postoperative complications

Some degree of bleeding after operation is usual, requiring routine use of wound drainage. On average about 50ml of blood drains during the first 24 hours. Serious haemorrhage may occur either from a slipped ligature or an overlooked divided vein, the most dangerous effect of which is pressure on the trachea by the accumulating blood. When respiratory obstruction caused by haemorrhage does occur, the wound should be reopened immediately in the ward. The patient is then returned to the operating theatre where the blood is removed and the bleeding point secured and the wound re-sutured.

Respiratory obstruction may also be caused by tracheal collapse, the accumulation of mucus in the trachea, laryngeal oedema or vocal cord paralysis or a combination of these causes. Simple tracheal suction may suffice to relieve the obstruction but bronchoscopy and, occasionally, a temporary tracheostomy may be necessary.

Postoperative tetany caused by removal or damage to the parathyroid glands is rare. When it does occur it can be controlled by the administration of calcium orally or intravenously (calcium gluconate), depending upon the severity of the clinical situation.

Postoperative thyroid crisis has almost disappeared as a clinical entity since the introduction of antithyroid drug preparation. If it should occur, sodium iodide, carbimazole, propranolol and hydrocortisone are drugs which may be used. Body cooling can be helpful in severe hyperpyrexia.

Late postoperative complications

Late postoperative complications of subtotal thyroidectomy are hypothyroidism, hyperthyroidism, chronic calcium deficiency and voice changes.

Hypothyroidism occurs in about 15 per cent of cases, it may be transient in some but in others it is permanent and will require treatment with thyroxine for life.

Hyperthyroidism is less common, occurring in about 5 per cent of cases. These patients should be treated with antithyroid drugs or radioiodine. A second operation should be avoided because of the technical problems posed by distorted anatomy; parathyroid gland and recurrent laryngeal nerve injury being much more likely.

Permanent hypoparathyroidism is best treated by the administration of calcium alone; long-term administration of Vitamin D may result in intoxication.

Some impairment of the voice may occur independently of recurrent laryngeal nerve damage, but is rarely of serious consequence and generally the voice returns to normal. In a few instances these voice changes (which may be caused by external laryngeal nerve injury) are permanent, but minor.

Index

Figures in medium type refer to page numbers; those in **bold** refer to figure and caption numbers.